the
HEALTHY
MOTHERHOOD
JOURNAL

ALSO FROM THE SEARS FAMILY LIBRARY

The Healthy Pregnancy Journal
The Healthy Pregnancy Book
The Baby Book
The Birth Book
The Breastfeeding Book
The Baby Sleep Book
The Attachment Parenting Book
The Portable Pediatrician
The Fussy Baby Book
The Family Nutrition Book
The Premature Baby Book
The A.D.D. Book
The Discipline Book
The Healthiest Kid in the Neighborhood
The Successful Child
The Dr. Sears T5 Wellness Plan
The Healthy Brain Book
25 Things Every New Mom Should Know: Essential First Steps for Mothers
25 Things Every New Dad Should Know: Essential First Steps for Fathers

the HEALTHY MOTHERHOOD JOURNAL

Practices, Prompts, and Support for Women in Baby's First Year

MARTHA SEARS, RN
HAYDEN SEARS DARNELL, MA
ERIN SEARS BASILE, MA

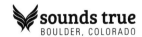
sounds true
BOULDER, COLORADO

Sounds True
Boulder, CO 80306

Published 2021

Book design by Karen Polaski
Illustrations © 2021 Mara Penny

Cover image by Mara Penny

Printed in South Korea

ISBN 978-1-68364-486-6

10 9 8 7 6 5 4 3 2 1

CONTENTS

WELCOME TO YOUR JOURNAL

Nearly everything about your life will change when you become a mother for the first time: your marriage, your priorities, your friendships, your career, your life goals, and even your very own body. You are a MOM now! It's a radically rich and fertile time in your life—and it calls you toward introspection, practically begging you to attend to self-care and self-reflection. The pages ahead are for you, for your journey into motherhood.

We developed *The Healthy Motherhood Journal* to guide new moms through new motherhood—with all the complexities, joys, challenges, sacrifice, and fulfillment this stage of life brings. By journaling, you will work through the beautiful chaos of new motherhood, keep your health on track, and create a keepsake that you can return to in years to come. Throughout the journal, we call on our experience as health advocates, parenting advisors, and nutrition educators to help you and your baby thrive. And when you thrive, your baby thrives.

This journal is unique, starting with its three contributing authors. Martha Sears, mother of eight grown children, grandmother of many, and now great-grandmother, brings the wisdom and perspective of age. Hayden Sears Darnell, mother of three tweens/teens, offers practical tools and important insight from one who is still on this motherhood journey. Erin Sears Basile, brand new mother, contributes her real and raw experiences with her new baby. These three Sears women combine their voices and different life stages to offer depth and breadth to your journaling experience.

Our hope is that this journal will help you connect with yourself on a deeper level and keep what's important at the forefront of your mind. By guiding you toward further self-awareness and understanding of your new role, the time you spend with this journal will help you blossom as a mother and woman. In these pages we will celebrate the unforgettable highs, magical moments, and mom wins, while also embracing the parts of motherhood that aren't as shareable—the fears, the worries, and the meltdowns (yours and Baby's). We want to create a space for all your feelings and experiences, and alongside these, provide insightful and often intimate prompts to encourage you to examine the full range of who you are and who you are becoming.

We welcome you to the new world of motherhood, and we look forward to guiding you with our collective experiences, acting as two older sisters and one eager-to-help mom. May you hold onto grace, patience, and peace as you embrace each moment and appreciate what it adds to your life.

With love and blessings,
Martha, Hayden, and Erin

A FEW TIPS TO GET STARTED

Each chapter in this journal is centered around a theme common to new motherhood: for example, your new identity, the journey of co-parenting, and your relationship with your baby. Every new mother's experience is different, so if a certain theme doesn't match where you are at, return to it when you are ready. And since each family's dynamic is unique, the questions and prompts can be adjusted to fit yours. This is your journal and your journey. We invite you to use it in any way that serves you best.

Since we know moms don't have ample hands-free writing time, we offer further questions to encourage you to go deeper in sections titled "To Ponder." These are prompts that you can simply spend time with as you go deeper within yourself. In each chapter you'll also find self-care check-ins, nourishment tips, and our favorite recipes to help you stay healthy. We offer frequent "moments for me"—collections of suggestions, meditations, and affirmations from our own mothering toolbox to help guide and support you. Each chapter ends with open space to create a tribute to yourself and all that you're learning.

We invite you to take a deep breath, settle in, and embrace how this journal can enhance your motherhood experience, guide your journey, and offer inspiration and support along the way. The opportunity to open yourself up to spiritual, emotional, physical, and mental growth is right here. Embrace YOUR version of motherhood.

The beauty of the written word is
that it can be held close to the heart
and read over and over again.

FLORENCE LITTAUER

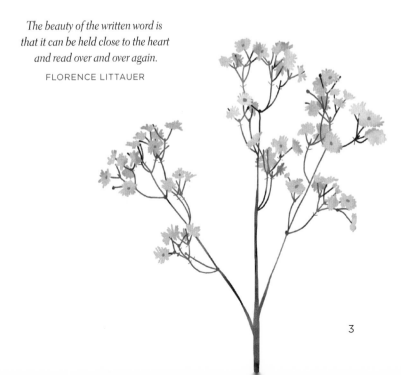

BECOMING A MOTHER

Congratulations! You have accomplished the most amazing and momentous feat nine months in the making. You are forever changed physically, mentally, emotionally, and spiritually. In light of all these changes, the contrasting nature of all you are feeling and experiencing may catch you off guard. You may be fluctuating between singing for joy and crawling into bed to cry; savoring each moment and wishing the day would end. You might feel like you are Superwoman one moment and Queen of Supertired the next. You may feel like you have finally found a piece of yourself and at the same time wonder if you have lost something central to who you are. You've likely never felt so fulfilled and empowered and so vulnerable at the same time.

Everything you are feeling is natural, honest, and real.

While the spotlight is on Baby, remember you have also given birth to yourself as a mother. Becoming a mother gives you an opportunity like no other to connect with yourself in a new and deeper way. Throughout this journal we will invite you to be present, responsive, and attuned to yourself as a woman who has become a mother and who is discovering aspects of herself that she never knew existed. This process of attuning and attaching first of all to yourself will in turn allow your baby to attach to you in a beautifully healthy way. As this process unfolds, you'll come to a fuller realization of yourself as a mother.

This chapter will guide you through unpacking the first days and weeks of stepping into motherhood. Whether your baby was born days or months ago, take some time to immerse yourself in that time and space. Allow your mind and heart to drift back and remember your incredible experience, capturing both the essence and the finer points of your journey so far. This time in your life is relatively brief, but it contains precious, poignant, and life-changing moments that will likely have a lasting impression on you—the woman you are and the mother you are becoming. This is YOUR time.

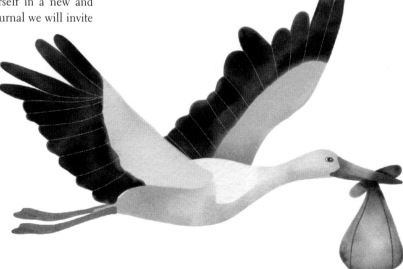

*Being a mother, as far as I can tell, is a constantly evolving
process of adapting to the needs of your child while also
changing and growing as a person in your own right.*

DEBORAH INSEL

What does "becoming a mother" mean to me?

_____

_____

_____

_____

_____

_____

_____

_____

_____

_____

_____

_____

_____

_____

_____

_____

_____

MY BIRTH STORY

Whether it's been a few days since your delivery or a few months, it's common for moms to replay their labor, delivery, and special moments that occurred during childbirth. The intensity of your experience wants your attention and reflection. There is no right way for your birth story—your initiation into motherhood—to play out. Some moms feel immensely proud of what they accomplished and are excited to share their story with everyone. Some feel like their experience was an intimately private one that they want to hold close. However you are feeling about it, there is a unique healing power to writing your birth story. It doesn't have to be tidy or eloquent; it can be as raw and deep as you are willing to go. Settle in, take a deep breath, and enjoy reliving this dual birthday—your baby's birth into the world and your birth as a mother.

_____

_____

_____

_____

_____

_____

_____

_____

TO PONDER

What feelings and emotions came up while writing my birth story?
What did I think my birth experience would be like?
What was it *actually* like? How do I reconcile the two?

A MOMENT FOR ME
Lens of Love Meditation

As you reflect on the events surrounding the miracle of birth, try to see yourself and the situation through the "lens of love"—a lens of grace and compassion. Birth is a remarkable experience full of expectations, unpredictable moments, and sometimes fear. As the hormonal roller coaster of this new season ebbs and flows, looking at everything that's happening through your lens of love will help you move from disappointment to peace.

Take a few moments to center yourself and focus on a slow, steady inhale and exhale. Allow any and all thoughts to arise. Notice those thoughts; celebrate the most joyous moment that comes to mind. Does any guilt or grief come up? Do any confusing thoughts arise? Are you hit with regret or feelings of inadequacy? Compassionately exhale those feelings and inhale healing and love. Take some time to record what came out of this meditation for you.

REFLECTING ON LABOR AND DELIVERY

Journaling through some of the more intense or unexpected moments of your initiation into motherhood will allow you to grow, laugh, remember, and have further appreciation for yourself and others involved. If your labor unfolded in a disappointing way, or in a way that surprised you, it will take some time to come to terms with it all.

Working though all your feelings here can help. Let this become your mantra: "I truly made the best decisions I could at the time for my baby and my body. I honor my body for every contraction, challenge, and victory. Every moment brought me closer to you, my precious Baby. I am a champion bringer-forth of life!"

What words or phrases came out of my mouth during labor
and delivery that were surprising or shocking?

_____

_____

_____

Humorous moments (reactions, jokes, mishaps . . .) that I just HAVE to remember:

_____

_____

_____

Were there special moments of support that I received (from my nurse,
partner, doula, or other labor support person) that had a huge impact?

_____

_____

_____

Was there a point in my labor when fear or panic set in?
Did unexpected challenges arise? How did I work through these?

_____

_____

_____

Do I have feelings of negativity or guilt regarding parts of my labor that need attention? How can I work through these feelings so resentment and blame do not set in? How can I show myself grace and forgiveness for what did not go as planned?

_____

_____

What did I learn about myself as a woman? What did I learn about myself as a mom?

_____

_____

Looking back, what would I want to say to myself at the beginning of labor?

_____

_____

TO PONDER

How did I connect with myself in a new way during my labor?
What did I learn about my strengths and areas of needed growth?
What did I learn about myself on a spiritual level?

A MOMENT FOR ME
A Place for Peace

Have you found a place in your home where you feel the most peaceful? On the roller coaster of emotions new motherhood brings, it's important that you can connect regularly to a serene space where you comfort yourself as you tend to Baby. Many moms love to have a rocking chair in the corner of the room, next to a window, to feed and comfort Baby—and also to comfort themselves. Natural light can help keep your mood up during the day, and a strand of twinkle lights can be soothing at night. It doesn't have to be the "perfect nursery," just a place to help foster feelings of peace. A place that sends an invitation to your mind, body, and spirit that it is time to relax from head to toe and soak in the love as you hold, rock, soothe, and feed your little miracle. If a physical place like this does not exist in your home, then create one in your imagination.

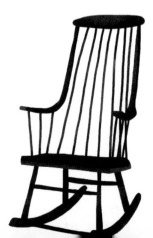

Self-Care Check In

On a scale of 1 to 10, where 1 means "really struggling" and 10 means "no problem":

What is my current stress level?

1 2 3 4 5 6 7 8 9 10

What is my current level of joy?

1 2 3 4 5 6 7 8 9 10

How am I doing on my self-talk/thought life?

1 2 3 4 5 6 7 8 9 10

Am I making nutrition and hydration a priority?

1 2 3 4 5 6 7 8 9 10

Am I managing my mental health?

1 2 3 4 5 6 7 8 9 10

Am I getting enough sleep and rest?

1 2 3 4 5 6 7 8 9 10

How am I doing at staying present?

1 2 3 4 5 6 7 8 9 10

Am I being supported in my mothering?

1 2 3 4 5 6 7 8 9 10

Am I making enough space for myself and my needs?

1 2 3 4 5 6 7 8 9 10

NOURISHMENT TIP
Feeding Station

In the first couple months of motherhood, it might seem like your baby is constantly eating and sleeping. You might feel liberated by this—or trapped. Either way, being prepared for marathon feeding sessions is key for your self-care. Your little angel is literally sucking the fluids out of you, and Mama needs to be filled with nutritious foods and plenty of water to best care for herself and baby. Having nutritious snacks and water at arm's reach where you typically feed Baby will help you to stay healthy. Here are tips for equipping your dual feeding station:

- A water bottle with a straw (aim for one day's total water of at least half your weight in ounces)
- Hydrating fruits and vegetables like cucumbers, melon, and berries
- One-handed foods like nuts (walnuts are great because they're high in omega-3 fatty acids, which are top fats for brain development)
- Foods that are high in B vitamins to help keep your energy up (Brazil nuts and sunflower seeds, for example)
- Dark chocolate–covered almonds (Mama needs some healthy treats too!)
- Phone charger
- Headphones
- Inspiring or funny podcasts
- Guided mediations
- Affirmation cards
- Lanolin nipple cream
- Burp cloth
- Nursing pillow
- Essential oil diffuser (many moms like peppermint, lavender, and citrus)

Lactation Cookies

- 3 cups organic old-fashioned rolled oats
- 1½ cups unbleached organic all-purpose flour or gluten-free flour
- 5 tablespoons brewer's yeast (a traditional aid for lactation)*
- 4 tablespoons hemp seeds
- ½ teaspoon baking powder
- ½ teaspoon baking soda
- 1 teaspoon ground cinnamon
- ¼ teaspoon salt
- ¾ cups organic unsalted butter
- 4 tablespoons unrefined organic virgin coconut oil
- 1 cup organic coconut palm sugar
- 1 large egg + 1 large egg yolk
- 2 teaspoons vanilla extract
- 1 cup dark chocolate chips/chunks

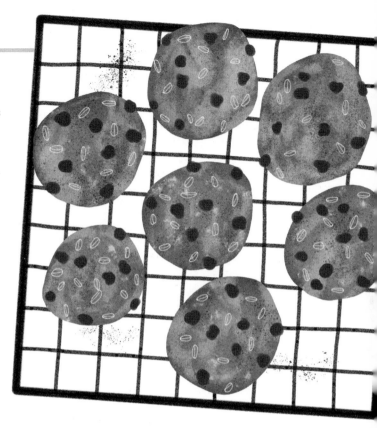

Heat the oven to 350°F.

In a medium bowl, whisk together the oats, flour, yeast, hemp seeds, baking powder, baking soda, cinnamon, and salt.

In a large bowl, beat the butter and coconut oil on medium speed until creamy. Add the sugar and beat on medium to high speed until fluffy. Add the egg and egg yolk and vanilla extract and beat until thoroughly combined.

Gradually add the dry ingredients to the wet ingredients, beating on low speed until just combined and mixed. Stir in the chocolate chips.

Scoop the dough into 1-inch rounds and place on a baking sheet about 2 inches apart. Bake for 10 to 14 minutes or until the bottoms are a beautiful golden brown.

Yields about 20 cookies

*Consider adding brewer's yeast to other food items like oatmeal, yogurt, smoothies, and muffins.

MEETING BABY

Meeting your child for the first time was likely at the forefront of your mind for many months of your pregnancy. Take some time now to immerse yourself in the anticipation of that incredible moment. It may seem like you will never forget such a special event, but these memories can easily fade as you move into your busy new life as a mother. You had months to get to know each other from the inside—you were not strangers. But that moment when you met Baby face to face may have left you awestruck. The hours after birth were a beautiful and complex mix of emotions, hormones, and vivid and even humorous moments. Take some time to dwell on, and record, how you said, "Hello, little person," in your own unique way.

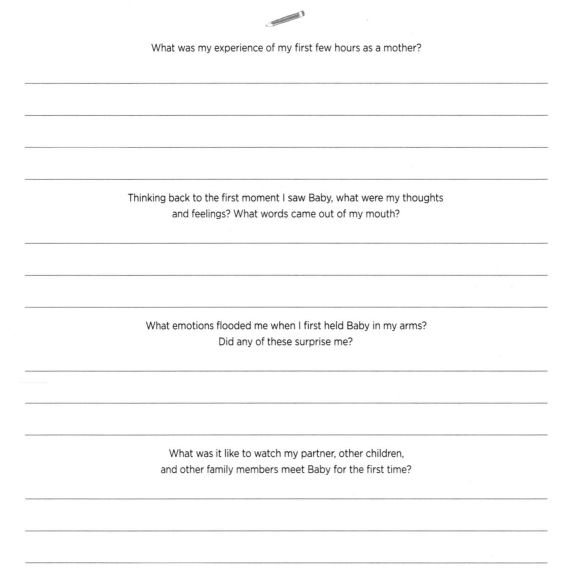

What was my experience of my first few hours as a mother?

_____

_____

_____

_____

Thinking back to the first moment I saw Baby, what were my thoughts
and feelings? What words came out of my mouth?

_____

_____

_____

What emotions flooded me when I first held Baby in my arms?
Did any of these surprise me?

_____

_____

_____

What was it like to watch my partner, other children,
and other family members meet Baby for the first time?

_____

_____

_____

Who were my first visitors? How did they support me? How did their presence, words, or energy recognize and celebrate me as a mother?

_____

_____

_____

Did I find myself wanting to share or keep Baby in my arms as long as possible? What was the first "mama bear" moment I remember?

_____

_____

_____

TO PONDER

Was there something about my baby that scared me?
In what ways did I recognize my baby?
In what ways did Baby feel like a stranger?

A MOMENT FOR ME
Connection Affirmation

I am secure and compassionately
   connected to all sides of my story.
I gave birth to a new woman in one
   profound moment of transformation.
I hold space for this new woman
   to strengthen and grow.
I nurture my soul with grace and honor.
I embrace the first precious moments
   with my baby as a priceless gift.
I will not be clouded or confused
   by external circumstances.
Time stands still and I soak in this
   pure, unconditional love.

My baby is perfect in every way and
   is an expression of my love.
I honor the mind, body, and soul
   connection with my baby.
With each breath, Baby and I will
   become more connected.
I look in my baby's eyes and hear her
   saying, "I love you, Mommy. You
   are the perfect mommy for me."
I feel Baby's breath rising and falling, and it
   reminds me to live in this moment.
In this moment I am content.

LETTING GO OF MY PREGNANT SELF

Before, you were two people in one body; now you are two people in two bodies. Do you miss being pregnant? Did you feel that there were perks that came with it? Perhaps you remember bursting into tears on day three postpartum because you suddenly realized you missed having that beautiful baby bump. Or maybe you miss being the center of attention now that all eyes are on your new baby. Feelings often come up that you can't prepare for and that may surprise you. This drastic shift from Baby in your womb to Baby in your arms brings about unique emotional, physical, and hormonal changes, and there is no right or wrong way to experience this transition.

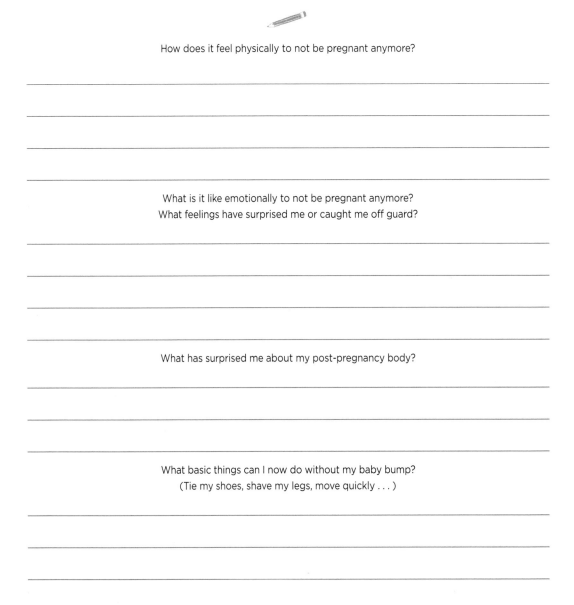

How does it feel physically to not be pregnant anymore?

_____

_____

_____

_____

What is it like emotionally to not be pregnant anymore?
What feelings have surprised me or caught me off guard?

_____

_____

_____

_____

What has surprised me about my post-pregnancy body?

_____

_____

_____

What basic things can I now do without my baby bump?
(Tie my shoes, shave my legs, move quickly . . .)

_____

_____

_____

What do I miss most, physically and emotionally, about having Baby inside me?

_____

_____

_____

_____

What was the first thing I ate, and what was the first
thing I did, that I couldn't while pregnant?

_____

_____

_____

_____

TO PONDER

Do I find myself eager to be pregnant again
someday, or am I relieved that it's over?
Did anything negative or traumatic happen during
pregnancy that needs to be worked through?
If so, how can I get support to do this work in a healthy way?

A MOMENT FOR ME
The Beginner's Mindset Meditation

Whether you are a first-time mom or have done this before, practice getting into a "beginner's mindset"—the awareness and understanding that each day (or even each hour) is a unique experience for you and your new family. Embracing a beginner's mindset allows you to let go of expectations and to experience each moment as it truly is: special, unique, magical, overwhelming . . .

Let the following mantra guide you: "I have a beginner's mindset, and I am free to feel and discover all the avenues of this new adventure. I accept my needs and my baby's needs for what they are today. I let go of the idea that I am going to be perfect and make space to show up as I am, knowing I am enough."

Final Reflections

The hand that rocks the cradle is the hand that rules the world.

WILLIAM ROSS WALLACE

Taking a moment to recognize and appreciate the new role I play in the world
now that I am a mom: In what ways do I feel more powerful and capable?

_____

_____

_____

_____

What did becoming a mother teach me or show me about myself
recently? How can I carry this lesson throughout my life?

_____

_____

_____

_____

What have I read, watched, or listened to recently that I want to remember?

_____

_____

_____

_____

What worries or fears about motherhood have I been able to work through?

_____

_____

_____

_____

What thoughts can I be mindful of that decrease my joy and peace, and
how can I best work through them and, if needed, get support?

_____

_____

_____

_____

How have I surprised myself or made myself proud as a mother?

_____

_____

_____

What do I want to let go of that is not serving me well?

_____

_____

_____

What would my future self want to say to me right now?

_____

_____

_____

A commitment, declaration, intention, or promise to myself moving forward
that helps me hold tight to what I have learned in this chapter:

_____

_____

_____

_____

A Love Note to Myself

Take some time to truly appreciate all that you are and all that you do for yourself, your baby, and those around you. Celebrate YOU in writing and memorialize the parts of yourself that deserve love and acknowledgment. Return to your words from time to time when you need a reminder.

Dear Me,

_____

_____

_____

_____

_____

_____

_____

_____

_____

_____

_____

_____

_____

_____

Draw, doodle, or attach pictures that describe
the essence of you becoming a mother.

2

YOUR NEW IDENTITY

Becoming a mother is one of the most profound transformations a woman will go through. Not only does a woman give birth to her baby, she also gives birth to herself as a mother. And with this comes new priorities, sensitivities, longings, and maybe even values. However, who she was doesn't vanish. Neither do her dreams, desires, need for creative outlets, or individuality. Still, wanting the best for your baby and helping your baby reach his or her full potential can be all-consuming, requiring you to stretch yourself and dig deep to access new strength. Giving your all for your baby must be balanced with making yourself a priority since your happiness will bring joy to the whole family. This will also help you avoid the dreaded "mommy burnout." We mother most beautifully and powerfully when we stay connected to ourselves and our intentions as our new identity blossoms.

Society sends us mixed messages about what mothering should look like, but the essence cuts across different cultures, socioeconomic status, and age groups. While every woman's experience of becoming a mother is different, many moms feel like they are going through an identity crisis of sorts. They love being with their children but also long to reclaim something within themselves that feels lost or far away. Yet many women find that in the long run, the fullness of who they become far outweighs the sacrifices. In the midst of late-night feedings, continuous snuggles, developmental challenges, and moments of mommy guilt that seem to deplete every ounce of your mental and physical energy, a profound transformation is taking place. Perhaps there is new strength and a deepening of self-love emerging. Perhaps having a baby is revealing aspects of yourself that you never realized you had.

Acknowledging your new identity brings with it a chance to embrace the highs and lows of this transformative time. Journaling through some of the most impactful aspects will help you embrace your new identity and feel confident that *you were made for this.*

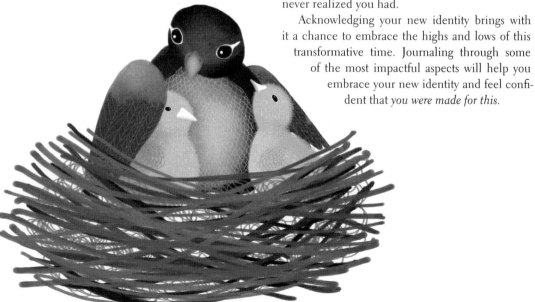

Love is not something we give or get; it is something that we nurture and grow, a connection that can only be cultivated between two people when it exists within each one of them — we can only love others as much as we love ourselves.

BRENÉ BROWN

What do I envision when I think about loving myself
through this incredible identity shift?

_____

_____

_____

_____

_____

_____

_____

_____

_____

_____

_____

_____

_____

_____

_____

THE GODDESS-MOM BOD

By now you have likely lived in your mommy body long enough to realize that you are a changed being not only emotionally and mentally but also physically, especially if this is your first baby. In a culture preoccupied with body image, it can feel automatic for us to be critical of our bodies and have unrealistic expectations. It's common to hear new moms long to "get my body back." Really look at what that is saying. How can we "get our body back" when we never lost it? In fact, we have gained a beautiful new physical form that has created a human life, which we are nurturing every single day. It's important to be mindful of the pressure to look a certain way because it can very much hinder the joy and confidence that comes with becoming a mom. Focusing on being healthy, not a certain shape or size, allows you to honor and respect your body. You can find balance by having appreciation and acceptance for your new-mom bod and all it has accomplished.

Where did my early programming of what a
woman's body "should" look like come from?

_____

_____

Have I struggled with body image in earlier parts of my life? How did I navigate that?

_____

_____

How has stepping into my new identity as a mother allowed for healing/growth in this area?

_____

_____

How have my ideas about or relationship with my breasts shifted since becoming
a mom? How has my partner's relationship with my body changed?

_____

_____

How can I shift any negative feelings I have about my body to feelings of appreciation?

_____

_____

Do I feel pressure to "lose the baby weight" or "get my body back"? If so, where is
the pressure coming from? (Myself, my partner, media, societal expectations . . .)

_____

_____

What about myself do I find beautiful and/or sexy? What
does my partner find beautiful or sexy about me?

_____

_____

_____

TO PONDER

Did I feel shame or negativity about my body pre-pregnancy? How
does that compare to how I feel now? How does my thought life
contribute to my body image? Who is a trusted friend I can lean
on as I work through what is holding me back in this area?

A MOMENT FOR ME
Reframing the "Baby Weight" Challenge

The human body is miraculous and mysterious. Consider the following factors and challenges your body must navigate in your day-to-day life. These will help you appreciate yourself and navigate challenges with grace as you're embracing your glorious mom bod.

SLEEP   Is Baby still waking up multiple times at night? (This is normal, by the way.) Frequent interruptions to deep sleep can throw off your metabolism.

STRESS   Cortisol, the stress hormone, can cause your body to keep extra pounds on.

BREASTFEEDING OR PUMPING   While this is in fact an awesome way to burn calories (about 300 per day, on average), many moms also share that they didn't lose those extra pounds until they were done breastfeeding. Think of it as nature's way of saying, "You are right where you're supposed to be, Mama." Embrace it!

MOVEMENT   Focus on the other advantages to exercise besides weight loss, like increased endorphins, better sleep, more energy, and a chance to release stress or worry while having fun with friends.

LETTING GO OF THE SCALE   Have you ever had a week when you felt like a wellness rock star, only to step on the scale and see a HIGHER number than you saw the week before? Talk about discouraging! Perhaps try putting the scale out of sight for a month and see how it goes.

CLOSET MAKEOVER   Go through your closet and find the clothes that make you feel amazing. Put those in the front.

TALK IT OUT   Choose a few friends you can be completely vulnerable with and courageously share your fears and struggles.

BE AWARE   Avoid getting sucked in by the "shoulds" that may pop up in your mind from mommy groups and the Internet.

HEALTH FROM THE INSIDE OUT   Pour love into your emotional, mental, and spiritual health.

I WAS MADE FOR THIS

You *were* made for this! You have the capacity to love and care for your baby even if you do not always feel like you do. Mentally, emotionally, and physically, you have what it takes to mother. Women have an innate awareness that enables us to nurture and care for our offspring. Our brains are even hardwired to attach to and bond with our babies. Yet motherhood comes more easily to some than to others. Some see motherhood as a calling, part of their contribution to the world, while other women may feel the opposite. Based on your life experience, you may need some support and modeling to help you ease into your new identity as a mom. Just remember, to your baby, YOU are the perfect fit. Imagine what your baby is thinking when he or she gazes into your eyes and gives you that special smile. Cherish *that* image of yourself.

Have I always wanted to be a mom? Is this a dream fulfilled, perhaps after a long time of trying, or was it a surprise?

_____

_____

In what ways do/did I feel prepared for this and in what ways not?

_____

_____

In what ways have my maternal instincts guided the attachment/bonding process?

_____

_____

What are some common "mom instincts" that I've noticed in myself? What has surprised (or shocked, or confused) me about them?

_____

_____

Have I had any "mommy tiger" moments yet? Tell that story.

_____

_____

_____

_____

Is there something specific to my (or my baby's) situation
that heightened a certain instinct in me?

_____

_____

_____

Who do I want to be as a mom? List some characters from books, movies, TV, or
your own daydreams who embody aspects of the mother you want to be.

_____

_____

_____

TO PONDER

Does an awareness of my maternal instincts give me
confidence and security? Does it ever frighten me?
Did this baby come after a loss? If so, have I created space
for the grieving process? How might I do this?

A MOMENT FOR ME
Postpartum-Friendly Movements

FREESTYLE DANCE PARTY   Bust out
your favorite upbeat songs and shake that
booty! Move in a way that feels free.

ELLIPTICAL MACHINE   If you are a gym-goer,
then this is the best low-impact cardio option since
it doesn't put too much pressure on your joints.

SWIMMING   Float and stroke your stress away.

YOGA   Try a beginners flow class, hatha,
or restorative yoga. Avoid power yoga or
heated yoga unless you had a strong practice
before Baby and feel ready to return to it.

RESISTANCE BANDS   These are great
for low-impact strength training.

WALKING   This is a great way to refresh
your mind as you renew your energy.

CORE   Try pelvic tilts, Cat/Cow
Pose, and Bridge Pose.

Self-Care Check In

On a scale of 1 to 10, where 1 means "really struggling" and 10 means "no problem":

What is my current stress level?

1   2   3   4   5   6   7   8   9   10

What is my current level of joy?

1   2   3   4   5   6   7   8   9   10

How am I doing on my self-talk/thought life?

1   2   3   4   5   6   7   8   9   10

Am I making nutrition and hydration a priority?

1   2   3   4   5   6   7   8   9   10

Am I managing my mental health?

1   2   3   4   5   6   7   8   9   10

Am I getting enough sleep and rest?

1   2   3   4   5   6   7   8   9   10

How am I doing at staying present?

1   2   3   4   5   6   7   8   9   10

Am I being supported in my mothering?

1   2   3   4   5   6   7   8   9   10

Am I making enough space for myself and my needs?

1   2   3   4   5   6   7   8   9   10

NOURISHMENT TIP
Choosing the "Right" Carbs

Caring for an ever-growing baby, let alone all the other household responsibilities, is a full-time job, so choosing your nutritional fuel is key. *Carb* may be a four-letter word, but carbs are also a key source of energy for keeping up with the little ones. Try to partner carbs with healthy fats, proteins, and fiber (like almond butter spread on apple slices). This helps the body absorb the sugar in a healthier way and keep energy levels more stable. Here are carbs that are "smart," meaning they have a low glycemic index, providing much-needed energy without the sugar crash.

- Quinoa
- Sweet potatoes
- Yogurt
- Apples
- Strawberries
- Peaches
- Whole grain or rye bread
- Soba noodles
- Wild rice
- Rolled or steel-cut oats

Build-Your-Own Trail Mix

Banana chips
Sunflower seeds
Pumpkin seeds
Walnuts
Almonds
Dark chocolate chips
Shaved unsweetened coconut
Brazil nuts
Dried pineapple
Dried cranberries
Dried cherries
Raisins
Pistachios
Dates

Simply choose your favorite
ingredients, mix them all up,
and divide into ¼ cup servings.

Choose two savory ingredients
for every sweet.

Buy raw nuts if possible,
and dried fruit with
no added sugar.

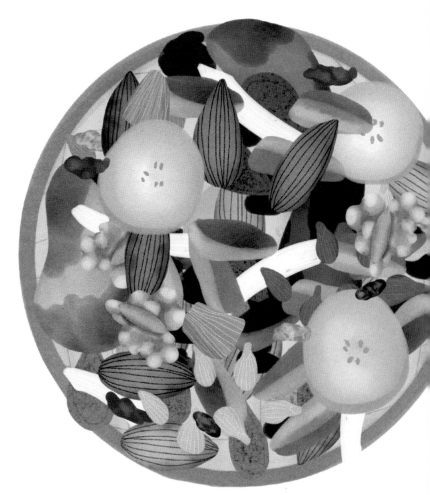

Burnout is a state of emotional exhaustion. A mom feels burnout when she has been out of balance for too long. With so much energy draining out of her, she reaches a point where she feels she has nothing left to give, yet her baby still needs her, and she must go on. She becomes unhappy, angry, and tired; she may start to question her ability to take care of her baby and blame herself for not enjoying motherhood. Women who find high value in being great mothers are at the greatest risk for burnout.

A number of factors can tip the balance toward burnout, such as having a high-needs baby, being in an unsupportive environment, navigating challenges within the marriage, having a sensitive soul, dealing with outside pressures, and fostering unrealistic expectations for parenting. Thinking you must "do it all" and not prioritizing your own well-being is a sure road to burnout. Perfectionism also sets new mommies up for failure. This is true even if outside appearances would suggest that "she has it all together," or others say, "I don't know how she does it." In our culture, being constantly busy equals succeeding, but at what cost? For most of us, this is an area that will need frequent attention and recalibration.

Based on what I know about my own energy levels and moods, what are some clues that I might be on the verge of burnout?

_____

_____

_____

How can I tell that I am on empty? What are some quick ways to refill my tank if I'm about to "lose it"?

_____

_____

How often do I feel burned out? What are some common contributors?

_____

_____

Knowing I can't do it all, what are my priorities?

_____

_____

Who/what can bring me the support that helps me avoid burnout?

_____

_____

What steps can I take to help myself recover from burnout?

_____

_____

_____

How does what I'm eating (or not eating) contribute to my well-being?

_____

_____

_____

TO PONDER

How does my burnout affect my baby and my partner?
How can I use this as motivation to stay in balance
instead of feeling shame about it?
Have I struggled in the past with burnout, or is this new for me?

A MOMENT FOR ME
Turning Perfectionism into "Good-enough-ism"

"I am not _____ enough." What words or phrases came to mind? Chances are good that whatever it was is not serving you. Getting stuck in negativity and "not-enough-ism" can make it extremely difficult to be productive and focused. Here are some examples of ways to live in a spirit of "good enough" and let go of all-or-nothing thinking. Think of these as mom hacks for getting through the day until you have more energy to give.

Think of *any* exercise as a victory, even
if it's "just" five minutes.
Let a clean-enough house be good enough. Let go
of the need for a perfectly tidy environment.

Maybe you only ate one vegetable
today. That's good enough.
Buy a store-bought meal (like rotisserie chicken).
No time to shower? At least wash your face
and put on some mascara or lip gloss, or
one thing that helps you feel pretty.
Baby won't sleep? Put her in a carrier and walk/
rock. Maybe you can get a nap out of it also!
Use a simple way to keep track of milestones
or memories, like an app or an email
address where you send quick messages to
yourself. The fancy baby book can wait.

LETTING GO

Embracing your new identity as a mother includes letting go—of plans, habits and routines, and expectations. Some life goals or dreams may need to shift to make room for your new reality. Entering this stage of life with an attitude of surrender can allow the mother in you to emerge more gracefully. When you don't hold so tightly to things like having a perfectly clean home, getting eight straight hours of sleep, taking a daily shower, sitting down to eat hot food, and defending the idea that time is your own, you will better be able to avoid resentment or feeling like a victim. For some things, this letting go might be temporary; for others, more permanent. Mourning the loss of both little and big things is important, and the complex feelings that come up may surprise you. Pay attention to them, and have compassion for yourself. Not only has this precious baby been born, but you were also reborn in a way. Your new reality won't always be easy, but it can bring with it an incredible opportunity to dig deep and access a new part of yourself. By letting go gracefully, you create space for new experiences to emerge.

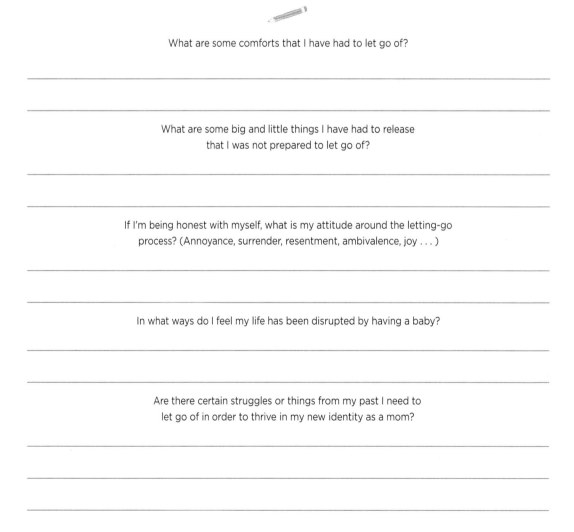

What are some comforts that I have had to let go of?

_____

_____

What are some big and little things I have had to release
that I was not prepared to let go of?

_____

_____

If I'm being honest with myself, what is my attitude around the letting-go
process? (Annoyance, surrender, resentment, ambivalence, joy . . .)

_____

_____

In what ways do I feel my life has been disrupted by having a baby?

_____

_____

Are there certain struggles or things from my past I need to
let go of in order to thrive in my new identity as a mom?

_____

_____

_____

Are there things I wanted to accomplish, and didn't, before starting
a family? How do I currently feel about them?

_____

_____

Do those around me have any expectations of me that I need to let go of?

_____

_____

TO PONDER

Did I have high hopes for having a boy or a girl? If so, how can I let go of
any lingering disappointment? Is there something I'm not willing to let
go of that I know I "should"? Is there an aspect to my identity that I feel
has been robbed from me? How can I navigate this intense feeling?

A MOMENT FOR ME
Confessions of a Recovering Perfectionist

"My dream had come true: I was finally a mom after a difficult journey. As long as I can remember, I have always dreamt of a beautiful life with my perfect family. While these dreams and visions weren't harmful in and of themselves, where I got into trouble was when challenges came and threatened my 'perfect mom' image. Like many moms, I fell into the 'I must do everything myself' mindset. I'll never forget the first day my husband went back to work after his paternity leave, and it was just Baby and me with no family members to turn to. The Supermom cape went on! I went about my day and was rocking it (so I thought), running errands, cleaning, and cooking. Until five o'clock hit. I was too tired to enjoy the dinner that I had spent so much time on, and I couldn't respond in a compassionate and patient way to my baby's needs. The quest for perfection had led me to extra stress and an inability to soak up the joy from my precious angel at bedtime. I had nothing left to give! I've since learned balance—asking for help, ordering takeout, and even just sitting and doing nothing. I listen to the quiet voice telling me to take off my Supermom cape before the burnout comes." (Erin Sears Basile, first-time mom)

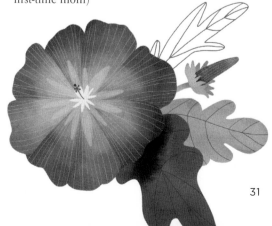

Final Reflections

I don't think perfect moms raise better kids,
I think good enough moms raise healthier kids.

LORI BREGMAN

How does this quote free me to mother from my true
identity and not a perfect version of myself?

_____

_____

_____

_____

What did becoming a mother teach me or show me about myself
recently? How can I carry this lesson throughout my life?

_____

_____

_____

What have I read, watched, or listened to recently that I want to remember?

_____

_____

_____

What worries or fears about motherhood have I been able to work through?

_____

_____

_____

_____

What thoughts can I be mindful of that decrease my joy and peace, and
how can I best work through them and, if needed, get support?

_____

_____

_____

_____

How have I surprised myself or made myself proud as a mother?

_____

_____

_____

What do I want to let go of that is not serving me well?

_____

_____

_____

What would my future self want to say to me right now?

_____

_____

_____

A commitment, declaration, intention, or promise to myself moving forward
that helps me hold tight to what I have learned in this chapter:

_____

_____

_____

_____

A Love Note to Myself

Take some time to truly appreciate all that you are and all that you do for yourself, your baby, and those around you. Celebrate YOU in writing and memorialize the parts of yourself that deserve love and acknowledgment. Return to your words from time to time when you need a reminder.

Dear Me,

_____

_____

_____

_____

_____

_____

_____

_____

_____

_____

_____

_____

_____

_____

Draw, doodle, or attach pictures that describe
the essence of you becoming a mother.

3

SURVIVING AND THRIVING
AS A NEW MOTHER

You prepared for motherhood physically by dutifully keeping your prenatal appointments, gathering all the things a baby needs, and loaning out your body for nine months while trying to stay healthy—not to mention keeping up with the duties you had before becoming pregnant. You prepared emotionally by daydreaming about holding your little one, working through fears, and managing the emotions that came with your body's changing hormones. You prepared mentally by reading books, making lists, picking out just the right name for Baby, and choosing the outfit you wanted Baby to wear home from the hospital.

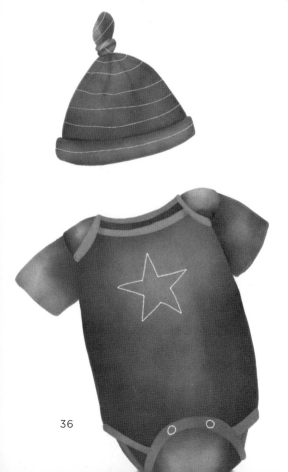

Perhaps you also had new spiritual stirrings that have drawn you to connect or reconnect to a power greater than yourself.

Settling into your new life as a mom happens on a day-by-day, go-with-the-flow basis; it's not something you can foresee and fully plan for, though it helps to think in terms of daytime and nighttime and the unique challenges each brings. Your daytime hours will be colored for a while with emotions you didn't know existed. The roller coaster of hormonal changes is one aspect of postpartum life that is completely beyond your control. Remember what it was like during early pregnancy? Only now the changes are often more sudden and more intense. And then there's nighttime—for most moms, the biggest challenge is that night is not what it used to be when you only had to answer to your own needs. It helps to accept that it will be a while before your baby gets the memo that the whole night is for sleeping.

Your task now is to not just *survive* but to *thrive* with your newborn. Some days it may seem like you are in survival mode, and other days you may find yourself being Supermom. Think of it as "sur-thriving"—this is the reality of any big change in life, including taking on your new role as mom.

You'll spend lots of time doing "nothing," just holding and nursing your baby. But time spent relaxing with your baby isn't really doing nothing. You're observing and learning, resting together, and settling in together.

WILLIAM SEARS

As I practice sur-thriving, what does doing "nothing" look like for me? What are some of the special moments of doing "nothing" that I want to remember?

_____

_____

_____

_____

_____

_____

_____

_____

_____

_____

_____

_____

_____

_____

_____

SETTLING INTO LIFE AS A MOM

The newness of birth has waned, the stream of visitors has dwindled, and now you get to settle into life with your baby. This can come with a mix of emotions that may feel difficult to articulate. One question every new mom gets is, "How is life with the new baby"? How about this for an answer: It's everything! You will experience each and every aspect of "sur-thriving." Some days you may wish that time would stop, and some days you may long for a new day. It can seem unbelievable how fast the weeks and months go by when each day feels like an eternity. Yet what a beautiful challenge to have! Clothing yourself each day with grace and patience can help manage expectations. Your experience is *your* experience. You and your baby are a unique expression of love in human form. Hold tight to this mommy mantra: "Today I will do my best, and that is enough," remembering that the definition of "my best" may look different each day.

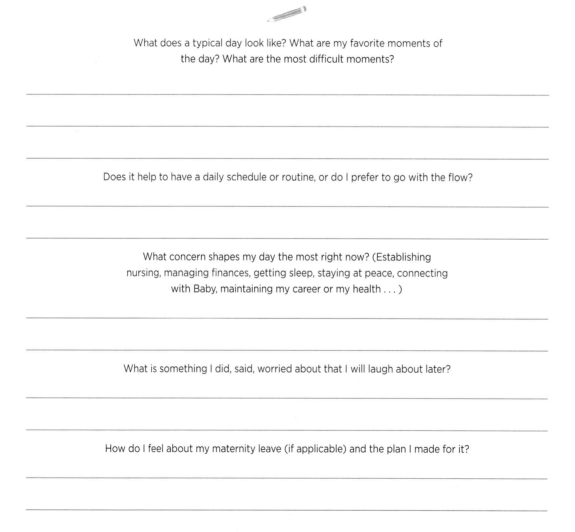

What does a typical day look like? What are my favorite moments of
the day? What are the most difficult moments?

_____

_____

_____

Does it help to have a daily schedule or routine, or do I prefer to go with the flow?

_____

_____

What concern shapes my day the most right now? (Establishing
nursing, managing finances, getting sleep, staying at peace, connecting
with Baby, maintaining my career or my health . . .)

_____

_____

What is something I did, said, worried about that I will laugh about later?

_____

_____

How do I feel about my maternity leave (if applicable) and the plan I made for it?

_____

_____

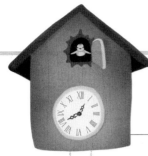

If my partner has/had family leave, how am I making/
did I make the most of that time?

_____

_____

What can I delegate to allow more room for me to thrive as a woman and a mother?

_____

_____

TO PONDER

If Baby could talk, how would he or she describe me?
(Joyful, stressed, content, in love, distracted, unsure, all of the above . . .)
Am I living my days with intention or am I mostly reacting
to my circumstances? What about my days can be
shifted so that I can move more into thriving?

A MOMENT FOR ME
Heathy Multitasking

Finding moments for self-care in your new role as a mother can be challenging. Here are tips from a first-time mom on building healthful habits into your daily routine with Baby:

"I remember around the one-month mark postpartum thinking to myself, *Wow, this really is a nonstop job!* I was ready to get back into a few of my daily exercise/movement and health habits, but the demanding schedule of a newborn definitely made that challenging. So, I chose small things to add throughout the day to help me get some movement in and also to remind me to check in with my emotional and spiritual wellness.
Sitting down and feeding the baby became a time to focus in on my breathing, with slow and even inhales and exhales through my nose, while visualizing a strong mantra, such as, 'I am peaceful, I am loved.'
I did calf raises while changing diapers—slowly raising up onto my toes and lowering back down.
While playing with Baby, I would squat up and down for some additional movement.
I would sing to my baby while walking around the house or neighborhood. Singing and moving help the brain produce endorphins.
I would listen to an empowering or funny podcast while doing household chores.
When it was possible, I would take a five minute 'mind mute,' simply relaxing in the beautiful moment of a quiet mind."
(Erin Sears Basile, first-time mom)

POSTPARTUM HORMONES AND ALL THE FEELS

The months following Baby's arrival are marked by a great deal of change in many areas. The hormones that supported your pregnancy and assisted you in labor have shifted into ones that help your body produce milk, help you communicate with your baby, and even shape the "new you" within. These hormones, along with the huge life changes that come during postpartum, can be overwhelming, and they can also change on a dime—often leaving Mom feeling confused. Most new moms experience mood changes ranging from mildly "blue" to full-blown depression; from tearful outbursts to utter rage; from boredom to complete hopelessness. This emotional volatility is often made worse by the belief that this "should" be one of the most joyful and anticipated times in a woman's life. Know that this is all normal, and hopefully you can meet all of the ups and downs with grace. Taking things one day at a time and letting go of the "shoulds" can help your mind and body find the freedom to ebb and flow during this unpredictable season of fluctuating hormones and all the feels.

In what ways do I see myself in the above statements?

_____

_____

_____

Describe some moments of unexpected heightened emotion.

_____

_____

_____

How have my environment and those around me been shaping my moods? Are there any shifts that need to be made?

_____

_____

_____

How am I managing/getting support for the more difficult feelings?

_____

_____

_____

What are my favorite ways to express the special and joyful moments?

_____

_____

_____

In what ways am I nurturing my spirit or inner thought life?

_____

_____

_____

TO PONDER

If I am being deeply honest with myself, am I being ruled by
my emotions and hormones? Do I have thoughts or feelings
that scare or concern me? How can I get support?

A MOMENT FOR ME
Building Your Mommy Tribe

Having a strong support system around you is key, especially during the early months. It's important to have people you can share with or vent to other than your family or partner. Receiving nourishment from strong female energy is especially vital during this time. There is nothing like the cosmic understanding that passes from mom to mom and encompasses everything you are feeling. Here are some ideas for where to find support:

La Leche League (for mother-to-mother breastfeeding support)

MOPS (Mothers of Preschoolers), a support group for moms with babies and toddlers

Free and local support groups organized through your local hospital or Facebook

Baby-and-me classes like yoga, stroller fitness, and music or story hour

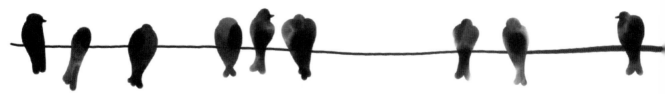

Self-Care Check In

On a scale of 1 to 10, where 1 means "really struggling" and 10 means "no problem":

What is my current stress level?

1   2   3   4   5   6   7   8   9   10

What is my current level of joy?

1   2   3   4   5   6   7   8   9   10

How am I doing on my self-talk/thought life?

1   2   3   4   5   6   7   8   9   10

Am I making nutrition and hydration a priority?

1   2   3   4   5   6   7   8   9   10

Am I managing my mental health?

1   2   3   4   5   6   7   8   9   10

Am I getting enough sleep and rest?

1   2   3   4   5   6   7   8   9   10

How am I doing at staying present?

1   2   3   4   5   6   7   8   9   10

Am I being supported in my mothering?

1   2   3   4   5   6   7   8   9   10

Am I making enough space for myself and my needs?

1   2   3   4   5   6   7   8   9   10

NOURISHMENT TIP
Iron

Iron is an essential mineral for women in general, and especially during postpartum (the suggested amount for women between ages nineteen and fifty is a minimum of 18 milligrams a day). This vital nutrient helps transport oxygen throughout the body and assists in energy production. Many women are iron deficient, so be sure to have your hemoglobin levels checked at your next medical appointment, especially if you had anemia during pregnancy. Here are some iron-rich foods to add to your diet:

- White beans
- Soy beans
- Lentils
- Spinach
- Tofu
- Kidney beans
- Red meat
- Pumpkin seeds
- Broccoli

Bonus—dark chocolate! Choose a bar with at least 45% cocoa and you get a whopping 7 milligrams of iron in a 3-ounce serving.

Crock-Pot Chili

  1 can kidney beans (rinsed)
  1 tablespoon coconut oil
  1 pound organic grass-fed ground beef or bison
1½ cups chopped sweet potatoes
  1 chopped green bell pepper
  1 cup chopped yellow onion
  2 garlic cloves, minced (or 1
     teaspoon garlic powder)
  2 bay leaves
  1 tablespoon chili powder
  2 teaspoons cumin
 16 ounces organic diced tomatoes (canned)
1½ teaspoons black pepper
     Salt to taste

In a large skillet, heat the oil over medium-high heat. Add the ground beef (or bison) and brown (about 5–7 minutes).

Cook the beef until no longer pink, then add it to the Crock-Pot.

Add the remaining ingredients except the salt. Cook for 8 hours on low (6 hours on high).

Before serving, stir in the salt to taste.

Serves 6

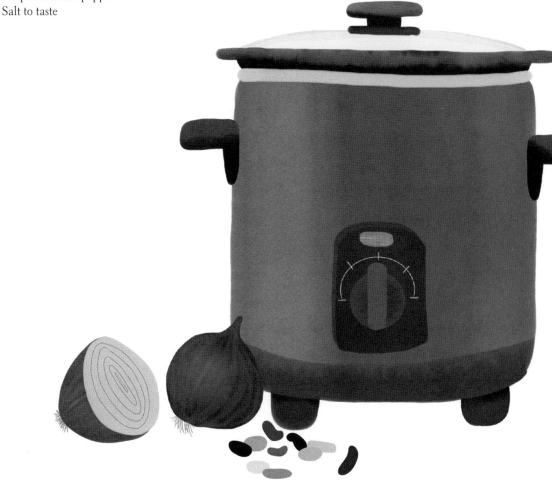

INTENTIONAL BONDING

One of the most treasured and perhaps mysterious aspects of life as a mother is the unbreakable bond that naturally develops between you and your baby. This happens at hormonal, emotional, physical, and spiritual levels. Some moms feel this bond innately and naturally settle into bonding practices that promote further attachment. Other moms may not feel this bond right away and need to be more intentional about creating connection. It's all normal and varies from mom to mom, even from pregnancy to pregnancy. As you connect with your baby, also connect with yourself in a new, more childlike way. Allow this season of life to bring you closer to yourself by cultivating a deep appreciation and love for all that you are and all that you are becoming.

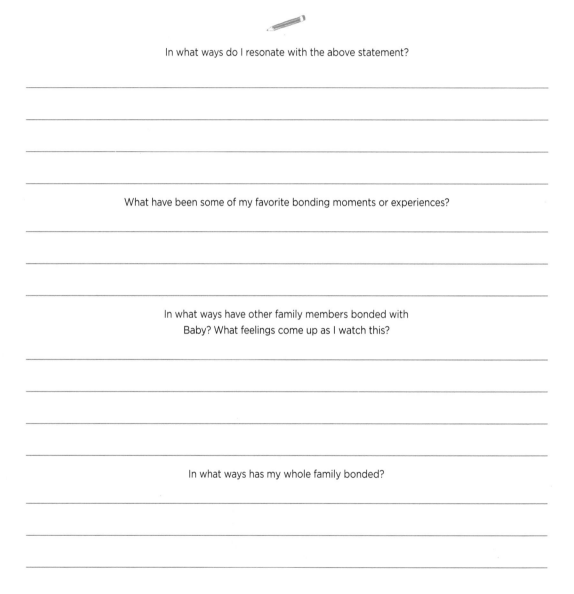

In what ways do I resonate with the above statement?

_____

_____

_____

_____

What have been some of my favorite bonding moments or experiences?

_____

_____

_____

In what ways have other family members bonded with
Baby? What feelings come up as I watch this?

_____

_____

_____

_____

In what ways has my whole family bonded?

_____

_____

_____

Did something happen that may have hindered our initial bonding? (Difficult birth, prolonged hospital stay, postpartum depression, breastfeeding difficulties . . .)

_____

_____

_____

Are there currently any distractions or situations that need to be recognized and addressed to better support bonding?

_____

_____

_____

TO PONDER

How has bonding with my baby allowed me to connect to myself
in a deeper way? What has the bonding experience taught me
about myself as a woman and as a mother? What childlike
desires to connect have I noticed stirring inside me?

A MOMENT FOR ME
Affirmation from Mom to Baby

Many moms have the "aha" moment sometime in the early months: I would do *anything* for my child. So why can it feel challenging to have the same devotion toward ourselves? Here is a peaceful bonding exercise to help you connect with Baby, and with yourself, before bedtime. The more you practice establishing a loving and grounding attachment to yourself, the more you can instill this in your baby.

As you're feeding or rocking your baby to sleep, attach an empowering word to each part of that little body. For instance, caress Baby's head and speak the word "calm," then move to Baby's heart and speak the word "compassion," then stroke Baby's hand and speak the word "gentleness," then place your hand on Baby's tummy and speak the word "healthy," and then brush Baby's feet and say the word "purpose." As you do this, you are subconsciously speaking these empowering words into your heart and mind as well!

Few things bring out feelings of desperation in the life of a new mother like sleep deprivation. The last month of your pregnancy, with the common nighttime discomforts, prepared you for having interrupted sleep as Baby woke frequently at night. But now, in the thick of it, nighttime mothering can seem to be all "survive" and no "thrive," which makes it even more important to take care of yourself and protect your sleep. In order to keep compassion for yourself and for Baby at the forefront of your mind, it's important to remember that it is common, and even healthy, for babies to continue waking at night for the first year or so for a variety of reasons:

growth spurts, teething, developmental stages, illness, even simply needing comfort (though some babies wake more frequently due to underlying reasons that should not be ignored). While helping baby sleep for longer stretches at night is a common goal, responding to Baby during the night is an important part of building a foundation of trust. Allow the time you have with Baby at night to be an enriching experience for both of you. There will be magical moments in the quiet of the night that will surprise you. To further explore sleeping solutions and options, see the recommended resources at the back of the book.

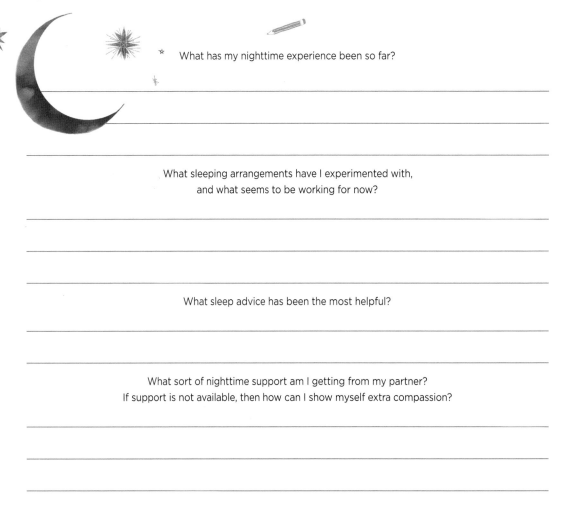

What has my nighttime experience been so far?

_____

_____

What sleeping arrangements have I experimented with,
and what seems to be working for now?

_____

_____

_____

What sleep advice has been the most helpful?

_____

_____

What sort of nighttime support am I getting from my partner?
If support is not available, then how can I show myself extra compassion?

_____

_____

_____

How has the nighttime experience affected me physically?

How is it making me feel about myself as a mother and a person?

_____

_____

_____

What magical nighttime moments do I always want to hold onto?

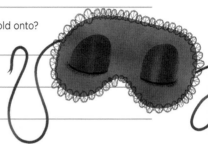

_____

_____

_____

TO PONDER

In the wee hours of the night, what unique thoughts and feelings come up? How can I use this time I have with myself and my baby for good? What am I consistently blaming or excusing because of my lack of sleep? How can I keep this in check?

A MOMENT FOR ME
A Healthy Mindset for Nighttime Parenting

"Utterly exhausted and so emotional today. I hear my mom friends say, 'It will get better,' but it doesn't feel like it. I want to believe them, but how does that help me today? Some days I just need to vent! I need to feel what I'm feeling—no judgment, just sit and feel. It does help knowing I'm not alone—I have a new cosmic connection to millions of women who have done this before me and have lived to tell the tale. I have such a profound love for my baby, but I am just so tired!" (Erin Sears Basile, first-time mom)

We hear you, Mama! Sometimes the unhealthiest thing we can do is put on a brave face and say, "I'm okay," when we are really struggling. We must feel to heal. This shift of mindset can help shed some grace and light on those moments of feeling hopeless. Many moms with babies who seem to need more at night have shared that finding some acceptance around where their baby is at has really helped. The following tips can help with this.

Stop looking at the clock at night

Remember that the baby is not
 waking up to irritate you

Recognize that Baby may be going through an
 important developmental stage or growth spurt

Soothe yourself as you are soothing Baby by
 saying a mantra or prayer out loud

Understand that each baby has
 different nighttime needs

Find ways to lighten your load and
 nourish yourself during the day

Final Reflections

*And the day came when the risk to remain tight in a bud
was more painful than the risk it took to blossom.*

ANAÏS NIN

What are the main things keeping me from fully blossoming
and thriving as a new mom and as a woman?

_____

_____

_____

_____

What did becoming a mother teach me or show me about myself
recently? How can I carry this lesson throughout my life?

_____

_____

_____

_____

What have I read, watched, or listened to recently that I want to remember?

_____

_____

_____

What worries or fears about motherhood have I been able to work through?

_____

_____

_____

_____

What thoughts can I be mindful of that decrease my joy and peace, and
how can I best work through them and, if needed, get support?

_____

_____

_____

_____

How have I surprised myself or made myself proud as a mother?

_____

_____

_____

What do I want to let go of that is not serving me well?

_____

_____

_____

What would my future self want to say to me right now?

_____

_____

_____

A commitment, declaration, intention, or promise to myself moving forward
that helps me hold tight to what I have learned in this chapter:

_____

_____

_____

_____

A Love Note to Myself

Take some time to truly appreciate all that you are and all that you do for yourself, your baby, and those around you. Celebrate YOU in writing and memorialize the parts of yourself that deserve love and acknowledgment. Return to your words from time to time when you need a reminder.

Dear Me,

_____

_____

_____

_____

_____

_____

_____

_____

_____

_____

_____

_____

_____

Draw, doodle, or attach pictures that describe
the essence of you becoming a mother.

4
NOURISHMENT

Having a new baby brought with it being pampered—with gifts, meals, and lots of help and attention. If only that could have lasted! Inevitably, things change, and meeting the needs of the baby, and the household, falls mainly on you. Proactively staying nourished will allow you to show up, full-power, for your family.

Perhaps at the forefront of a mom's mind is feeding her baby. The countless moments you spend feeding your baby will likely include some of the most special and cherished memories to hold onto. Still, all this feeding can be taxing to your body. If you are finding the constant feeding or pumping schedule exhausting, know that you are not alone! You are keeping another human alive, which is a huge deal, so celebrate that even, and especially, if the feeding relationship has been rocky or different than you envisioned. Experimenting with what feeding positions help you feel the most connected and relaxed will enhance the experience for both of you.

Because your body is so important to your feeding baby, what you feed yourself is important, too. During pregnancy you may have paid close attention to what went in your mouth. Many pregnant moms step up their nutritious eating and are extra disciplined to minimize health-sabotaging junk food. Continuing this effort now is just as important, and it will also assist in your physical recovery from pregnancy and birth. Nourish yourself with plenty of fresh fruits and veggies, lean proteins, healthy fats, and lots and lots of water. Keeping your kitchen stocked with quick and easy-to-grab healthy snacks and meals will help you avoid the junk food spiral—although there is no harm in keeping a few of your favorite treats on hand!

When some people hear the word "nourishment," they only think of food. Yet just as there are foods that are nourishing to our bodies and foods that are not, there are better and worse ways to nourish ourselves mentally and emotionally. Just as junk food is toxic to your body, toxic thoughts and words are damaging to your life and can permeate your experience of motherhood, intensifying feelings of being overwhelmed and "not enough." Practice cultivating a healthy thought life with positive self-talk and gratitude. Surround yourself with thoughts, sounds, images, and people who nourish you physically and emotionally and who bring you peace. What Mom and Baby need the most is a nourishing and compassionate environment to help the feeding relationship thrive.

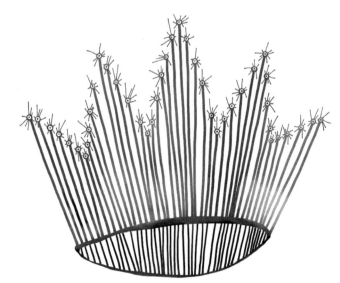

Sometimes while caring for my baby,
I wish someone would care for me that way.

MARTHA SEARS

In what ways do I deeply long to be nurtured and
cared for as a mother would care for her baby?

_____

_____

_____

_____

_____

_____

_____

_____

_____

_____

_____

_____

_____

_____

_____

_____

_____

QUEEN AND COW

The hormones released during breastfeeding are a special superpower for moms—oxytocin helps facilitate bonding and prolactin has a relaxing effect. Studies show that these hormones support breastfeeding moms to have less postpartum anxiety and depression. Whether you're breastfeeding or bottle feeding, nourishing your baby is likely one of your top concerns right now, and it's what you spend much of your time and energy doing. Sometimes, with nonstop feedings and feeling physically drained, you may see yourself as a cow (just keeping it real!). But there are also moments when you feel like the queen of your realm, with the uniquely powerful ability to nurture and nourish your baby. The blessings of motherhood encompass these seemingly opposite feelings, cow and queen, and that is the reality of being Mom.

What has my experience of feeding Baby been like? What was most unexpected?

_____

_____

_____

_____

What about nourishing my baby makes me feel like a queen?

_____

_____

_____

What about feeding my baby gets me feeling like a "mama cow"?

_____

_____

_____

What were some struggles around feeding Baby, and how did I navigate them?

_____

_____

_____

What have been my favorite resources and sources of support for feeding?

_____

_____

_____

What are some special and/or funny things my partner has said about feeding Baby?

_____

_____

_____

Are there feeding positions that I find more restful for me? More efficient for Baby?

_____

_____

_____

TO PONDER

Does feeding my baby ever bring up feelings of resentment or other
negative feelings toward Baby or myself? How have my life experiences
influenced my feelings and decisions about nourishing my baby?

A MOMENT FOR ME
New-Mommy Mantra

"I embrace my cherished mom bod. This body housed and birthed a human being. This body is to be celebrated. This body is not to be shamed. I honor every bump and scar, and I will proudly wear whatever clothing size I am. I will have patience and compassion for myself as I recover and let go of any pressure to 'lose the baby weight' in a way that is less than healthy. Right now, in this moment, I am how I am meant to be. I accept and value that I am both a beautiful mama queen, matriarch of my home, AND a giver of life with the superpower to nourish my baby. I honor and celebrate all aspects of myself."

NOURISHING YOU

To be able to nourish your baby, you must first be well-nourished. It is common for new moms to put their needs on the back burner because they feel like they don't have the time to invest in their own healthy eating. Yet eating nutritious food is vital for thriving as a new mom and important for your long-term health, vitality, and happiness. While it will take some time and intention, investing in yourself is worth it—don't miss out on the valuable support that good nutrition can provide. (If you need guidance in the area of nutrition, see our recommended resources in the back.)

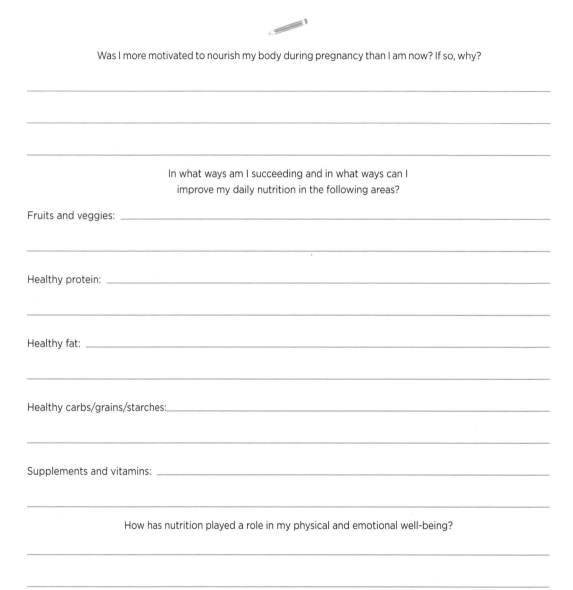

Was I more motivated to nourish my body during pregnancy than I am now? If so, why?

_____

_____

_____

In what ways am I succeeding and in what ways can I
improve my daily nutrition in the following areas?

Fruits and veggies: _____

_____

Healthy protein: _____

_____

Healthy fat: _____

_____

Healthy carbs/grains/starches:_____

_____

Supplements and vitamins: _____

_____

How has nutrition played a role in my physical and emotional well-being?

_____

_____

What obstacles keep me from choosing healthy food and getting enough to eat? (Lack of time, not knowing what to eat, not having quick and easy options available, needing more help . . .)

_____

_____

_____

Besides food, what other things give me a sense of nourishment? (Fresh air, music, movement, physical touch, nature, scripture, poetry . . .)

_____

_____

_____

TO PONDER

What was my relationship with food like before Baby?
Are there any shifts that I want to make for long-term health?
Do I often lean on food for nourishment when another
nourishing activity would be a healthier choice?

A MOMENT FOR ME
Motherhood Support

What new moms need to truly shine is support. When people offer to help, TAKE THEM UP ON IT!!! Even if it's been months since Baby arrived, allow others to serve you. Here are some ideas for how to do this:

Have people bring their favorite healthy freezer meal (like the vegetable lentil soup you'll find a recipe for later in this chapter)

Have someone assemble a quick grab box of snacks (trail mix, nuts, seeds, hard boiled eggs, single-serve guacamole and hummus packets, Greek yogurt, fruits and veggies, coconut water, dark chocolate, lactation cookies, energy bars)

Ask for grocery delivery gift cards

Organize a meal train where people bring meals

Request a gift card for a mani-pedi or massage and a friend to be on baby duty

Hire a weekly "mommy's helper" to assist with household duties like cleaning and laundry

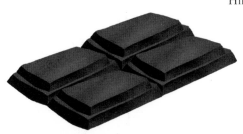

Self-Care Check In

On a scale of 1 to 10, where 1 means "really struggling" and 10 means "no problem":

What is my current stress level?

1   2   3   4   5   6   7   8   9   10

What is my current level of joy?

1   2   3   4   5   6   7   8   9   10

How am I doing on my self-talk/thought life?

1   2   3   4   5   6   7   8   9   10

Am I making nutrition and hydration a priority?

1   2   3   4   5   6   7   8   9   10

Am I managing my mental health?

1   2   3   4   5   6   7   8   9   10

Am I getting enough sleep and rest?

1   2   3   4   5   6   7   8   9   10

How am I doing at staying present?

1   2   3   4   5   6   7   8   9   10

Am I being supported in my mothering?

1   2   3   4   5   6   7   8   9   10

Am I making enough space for myself and my needs?

1   2   3   4   5   6   7   8   9   10

NOURISHMENT TIP
Fiber

Your digestive tract may take a while to adjust as your organs shift back into pre-baby position (many women find constipation to be an issue postpartum). Eating plenty of fiber is key to finding your new normal. The good news is, if you're eating a healthy and balanced diet that is rich in real, whole foods, you most likely are already getting plenty of fiber. Foods high in fiber include black beans, sweet potatoes, broccoli, lentils, oatmeal, and green leafy veggies. Aim for 25–30 grams per day. And remember, eating a lot of fiber but not drinking enough water will backfire. Aim for drinking at least an ounce of filtered water per pound of half your body weight.

Vegetable Lentil Soup

    Large onion, diced
3 carrots, diced
3 stalks of celery, diced
1 red bell pepper, diced
1 tablespoon olive oil
    28-ounce can organic fire-roasted tomatoes
32 ounces of vegetable broth
8 ounces of water
2 cups of dried lentils
2 yellow potatoes, diced
2 zucchinis, diced
1 cup green beans, diced
1 cup kale or Swiss chard, chopped
1 tablespoon Italian parsley, chopped
1 teaspoon dried basil
1 teaspoon dried oregano
2 bay leaves
1 teaspoon dried thyme
    Salt and pepper to taste
3 tablespoons nutritional yeast (optional)

Sauté the onion in olive oil until slightly soft. Add the carrots, celery, and red pepper, and sauté until soft.

Add the tomatoes, broth, lentils, dried herbs, salt, and pepper. Bring to a boil and then simmer (lid tilted) for about 20 minutes.

Then add the potatoes and simmer for 5 to 10 minutes (covered).

Add the zucchini, green beans, kale or chard, and parsley, and simmer again until desired tenderness (about 15 minutes).

Add the nutritional yeast at the end and season with salt and pepper to taste.

Serves 6

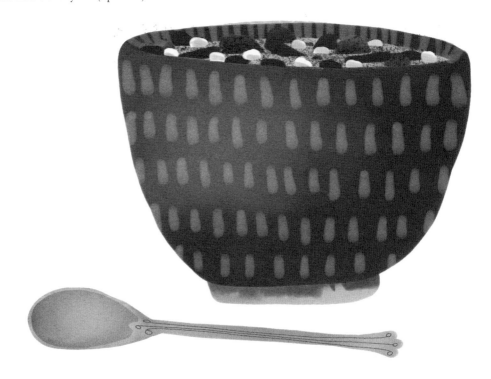

RECOVER, HEAL, STRENGTHEN

Physical recovery from pregnancy and birth is an ongoing process that can take many months. From stretch marks to sex, being a mother comes with a new physical reality. You can find a balance between having patience with the process and intentionally investing in your physical health, recovery, and nourishment. Just as each pregnancy and birth is unique, each recovery is, too. For example, some couples may be ready for lovemaking after six weeks, yet for some it might take much longer. Other factors, like sleep (or lack thereof, we should say), hormonal swings, scars from surgery, lack of self-confidence, and stress can make physical intimacy and recovery more of a challenge. "Progress, not perfection" can be a valuable mantra while your body heals and strengthens. Compassion—with yourself and your partner—during the process is a valuable form of nourishment to give yourself.

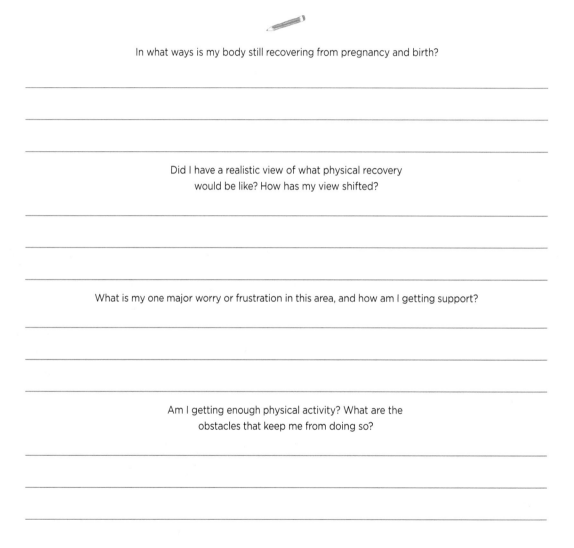

In what ways is my body still recovering from pregnancy and birth?

Did I have a realistic view of what physical recovery
would be like? How has my view shifted?

What is my one major worry or frustration in this area, and how am I getting support?

Am I getting enough physical activity? What are the
obstacles that keep me from doing so?

In what ways do I struggle with comparison and pressure from social
media, those around me, and myself regarding my body?

_____

_____

_____

In what ways do I feel stronger now than I felt before I became pregnant?

_____

_____

_____

TO PONDER

What are the ways I'm physically able to connect with my partner
that bring me a sense of nourishment? Do I feel a sense of obligation
or negativity around my physical limitations postpartum?

A MOMENT FOR ME
Healing After Baby

The birth process gave you a beautiful baby, but a weakened pelvic floor came along for the ride. Here are some gentle movements for strengthening the pelvic floor that you can weave into your day.

KEGEL BREATHS   Breathe in and engage the pelvic floor muscles (this should feel like you're trying not to pee). Hold for ten seconds, then relax. Build up over time to ten reps.

KEGEL BRIDGE   Lie on the floor with your knees bent and palms by your hips. Breathe in and engage your pelvic muscles; then lift your hips slightly. Hold for ten seconds, then relax. Work up to ten reps over time. If Baby needs playtime, have her sit on your belly. Babies make great personal trainers and cheerleaders!

BELLY BREATHING   This can be done whenever, wherever. Simply sit, stand, or lie down, and completely relax your abdominal muscles as you inhale (like you're inflating a balloon). Then, engage your pelvic floor muscles and abdominal muscles as you exhale by drawing in your belly button (deflating the balloon). You can alternate a smooth, slow breath and a more vigorous, pulsing breath, saying "hut" as you exhale forcefully.

POSTURE   While standing, tuck your chin in to elongate your neck. Then pull your shoulders down and back, and tighten your abdominal muscles while pulling your belly into your backbone. Tighten that pelvic floor and practice Kegels.

SELF-APPRECIATION AND GRATITUDE

With a little one to pour all your energy into, it's easy to ignore your inner life. While you can and should look to others for nourishment, appreciation, and a sense of purpose during this time, it's also important to be able to offer these to yourself. There is a security that comes from not having to rely solely on others for your sense of well-being. Our thoughts set the tone for how we live and how we treat ourselves and others, directly affecting who we become. Being intentional about appreciating yourself and showing yourself gratitude does not always come naturally, so it may take some practice. This practice is well worth the time and effort, though, because it can help combat resentment, depression, and self-doubt. Be gentle with yourself, Mama: it will help you to be gentler with your baby and those around you.

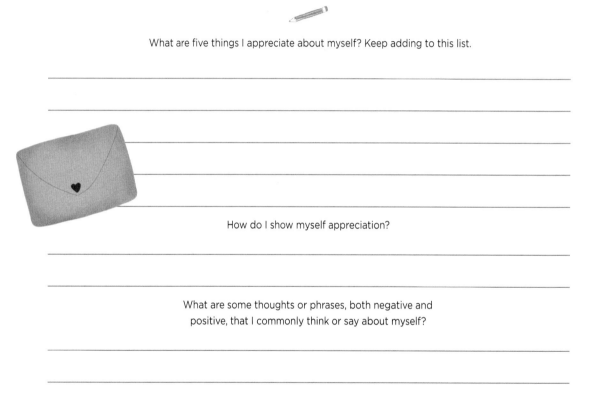

What are five things I appreciate about myself? Keep adding to this list.

How do I show myself appreciation?

What are some thoughts or phrases, both negative and
positive, that I commonly think or say about myself?

How can I reframe the negative thoughts and phrases so that they are helpful
and not harmful? For example, "I can't do this anymore" can turn into "One day
at a time." "I'll never sleep again" becomes "Things won't always be this way."

What are five things that I am grateful or thankful
for? Consider adding to this list frequently.

_____

_____

_____

_____

_____

In what ways do I have a new appreciation for my own mom?

_____

_____

_____

TO PONDER

Are there things that have been said to me that I have internalized
and replay in my mind, and that distract me from self-appreciation?
Who around me gives me positive messages about myself that I
can hold onto when I'm struggling with self-gratitude?

A MOMENT FOR ME
Self-acceptance Affirmation

I am strong. I am beautiful. I change the world one day at a time by being a mom. I am enough. I honor my body exactly as it is today. Today I will nourish my body with nutrition, nourish my mind through positive self-talk, and nourish my soul by finding the message in the "mess." I will not fall into the "getting my body back" trap. My body never left. It's different and I'm different, and that's okay—I don't want to be who I was before I had my baby, because my baby made me a stronger version of myself, inside and out. My body made me a mother.

Final Reflections

The child, in the decisive first years of his life, has the experience
of his mother as an all-enveloping, protective, nourishing power.
Mother is food; she is love; she is warmth; she is earth. To be
loved by her means to be alive, to be rooted, to be at home.

ERICH FROMM

Taking a moment to truly appreciate all that I am and all that I give my
baby: How can I channel that love and nourishment toward myself?

_____

_____

_____

_____

What did becoming a mother teach me or show me about myself
recently? How can I carry this lesson throughout my life?

_____

_____

_____

What have I read, watched, or listened to recently that I want to remember?

_____

_____

_____

What worries or fears about motherhood have I been able to work through?

_____

_____

_____

_____

What thoughts can I be mindful of that decrease my joy and peace, and
how can I best work through them and, if needed, get support?

_____

_____

_____

_____

How have I surprised myself or made myself proud as a mother?

_____

_____

_____

What do I want to let go of that is not serving me well?

_____

_____

_____

What would my future self want to say to me right now?

_____

_____

_____

A commitment, declaration, intention, or promise to myself moving forward
that helps me hold tight to what I have learned in this chapter:

_____

_____

_____

_____

A Love Note to Myself

Take some time to truly appreciate all that you are and all that you do for yourself, your baby, and those around you. Celebrate YOU in writing and memorialize the parts of yourself that deserve love and acknowledgment. Return to your words from time to time when you need a reminder.

Dear Me,

_____

_____

_____

_____

_____

_____

_____

_____

_____

_____

_____

_____

_____

_____

_____

Draw, doodle, or attach pictures that describe
the essence of you becoming a mother.

5

MOTHER, AND PARTNER

It's amazing how such a little being can have such a dramatic effect on the household. Whether you are a first-time parent or new to the world of multiple kids, you were once parented, and perhaps you are already getting a taste of the complexities. No matter how much you have prepared for life as a mother, much can only be learned on the fly, in the day-to-day of parenthood, and it can seem like the job description gets written as you go. Yet there's plenty we can learn and plan for through understanding our family of origin.

Exploring your family of origin is an important part of understanding how you will parent your own child. And getting insight into your partner's family of origin will help you understand the dynamic the two of you are creating. For most couples, this is a mosaic of both parents' experiences along with each partner's own ideas about what they both want for their family. For the two of you, identifying the healthy and unhealthy aspects of how you were parented is important so that you can intentionally leave behind what is not going to serve your family and make sure to preserve what is.

Based on your personality, your baby's temperament, your family of origin, your life experience, and with whom you surround yourself, your parenting style will develop. While it is valuable to explore resources (our favorite resource is the organization Attachment Parenting International), it's important to remember that you already have everything you need to be what your baby needs. Your own, unique intuition will be your most trusted guide to what is best for you and your baby.

In fact, sometimes advice and opinions, while well-meaning, can undermine your confidence in yourself as a mother since they may contradict or disagree with what you think is best. If this sounds overwhelming, take a deep breath and trust that you and your baby will work things out one step at a time.

Dads often have different approaches to parenting (it can come more naturally to moms for many reasons). Allowing Dad to be a dad and find his unique ways can help unify the partnership and make co-parenting more successful and more enjoyable. Journaling through the complexities of co-parenting will provide insight and help you further connect with yourself as your motherhood journey unfolds. Since everyone's situation is different, as you're going through this chapter feel free to adjust the questions to fit your co-parenting dynamic.

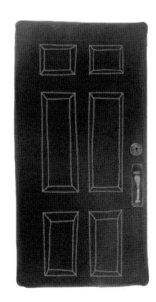
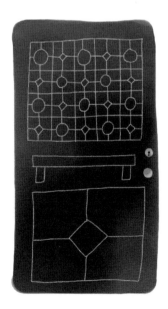

The Family—that dear octopus from whose tentacles we never
quite escape, nor, in our inmost hearts, never quite wish to.

DODIE SMITH

In what ways have I found new value in having a life partner during this season of life?

_____

_____

_____

_____

_____

_____

_____

_____

_____

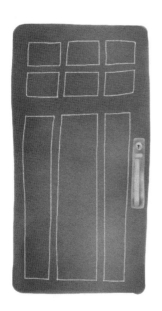 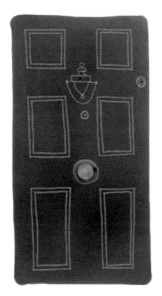 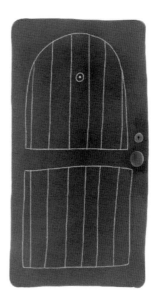

Do you remember what it was like to be just the two of you? Becoming parents is likely the most profound thing that will happen to you as a couple and can bring with it feelings of elation, completion, and purpose, giving your life new meaning. On the other hand, a couple can feel overwhelmed, confused, and ambushed as they try to find a new rhythm that includes Baby. Parenthood brings with it the potential to unify or divide, and most couples experience a bit of both—and this is a natural part of the journey. As you are developing as a mom, remember your partner is also experiencing this transition in a unique way. Some moms find it challenging to put faith in their partner and allow them to grow as a parent. Co-parenting is based on trust and support, and making room for both is important and rewarding. It can be easy to focus all your attention on Baby, but be sure to keep the relationship with your partner a priority. While it may be hard to envision now, someday it will just be the two of you again.

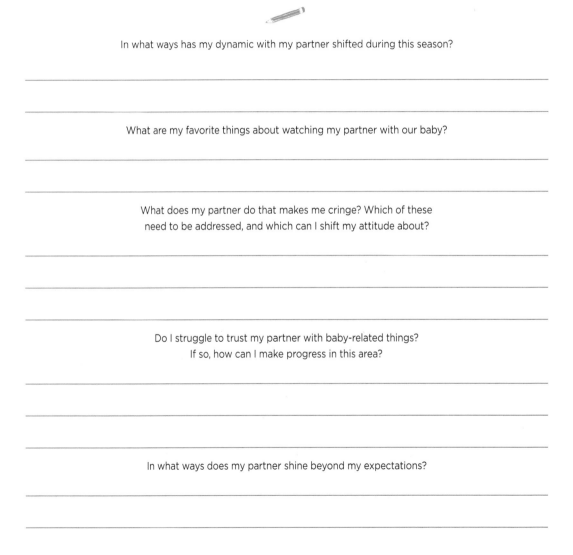

In what ways has my dynamic with my partner shifted during this season?

_____

_____

What are my favorite things about watching my partner with our baby?

_____

_____

What does my partner do that makes me cringe? Which of these
need to be addressed, and which can I shift my attitude about?

_____

_____

_____

Do I struggle to trust my partner with baby-related things?
If so, how can I make progress in this area?

_____

_____

_____

In what ways does my partner shine beyond my expectations?

_____

_____

What have I learned about myself so far as I have experienced co-parenting?

_____

_____

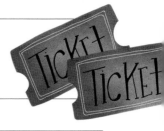

What are some activities I'm looking forward to doing, or
getting back to doing, with just my partner?

_____

_____

How am I feeling about physical connection and sex with
my partner? How does my partner feel about it?

_____

_____

TO PONDER

Do I have any fears or negativity around the topic of sex?
How can I work through these with my partner or a trusted confidant? Are
there issues between me and my partner that we have put off addressing?
How can I take healthy steps toward resolving these?

A MOMENT FOR ME
Guided Trust Meditation

Showing up for a relationship in a healthy, authentic way starts with integrating your own head and heart. The clearer you are—with yourself and with your partner—about your wants and needs, the clearer the path to a healthy partnership. When relationship and co-parenting challenges arise, here is a guided meditation to help. But first:

1 Quiet your mind: connect with your breath through a slow and steady inhale and exhale.

2 Honor and accept any "mama bear" or difficult thoughts and emotions with zero judgment.

3 Notice if those thoughts and emotions are coming from love or fear.

"I embrace every part of my mama-bear soul. I trust my intuition. I am doing the best I can. I am strong. I am capable of being the mom my baby needs me to be. My wants and needs are valid. I react and respond to my partner out of love. I have compassion for my partner. I trust my partner. Together we will do what is best for our baby."

MOTHER, AND PARTNER   71

FAMILIES OF ORIGIN

Who you are as a person, for better *and* worse, was significantly influenced by your family of origin and how it functioned. Since your childhood affects your relationships, it's necessary to explore that dynamic to understand yourself (and your partner) and how you will work together as co-parents. Examining how your parents communicated, their values and faith, and how they showed emotion and love will give you huge insights into where you will be successful and where you will struggle and need healing and support. Keep in mind that this is an ongoing process; different seasons in your family's life will allow more to surface and be explored. Your family of origin can also shape your idea of what your own family experience will be like. For instance, someone from a large family has a different image of family life than someone who is an only child. Neither one is right or wrong, just different. Celebrate that, and use this exploration as an opportunity to connect more fully with yourself and with your partner.

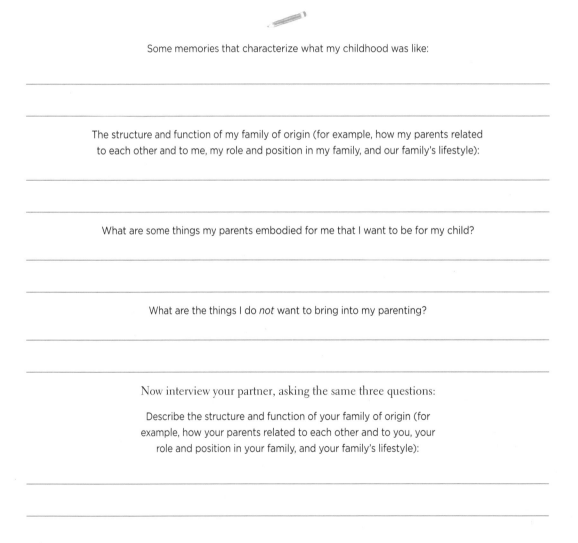

Some memories that characterize what my childhood was like:

_____

_____

The structure and function of my family of origin (for example, how my parents related to each other and to me, my role and position in my family, and our family's lifestyle):

_____

_____

What are some things my parents embodied for me that I want to be for my child?

_____

_____

What are the things I do *not* want to bring into my parenting?

_____

_____

Now interview your partner, asking the same three questions:

Describe the structure and function of your family of origin (for example, how your parents related to each other and to you, your role and position in your family, and your family's lifestyle):

_____

_____

What are some things your parents embodied for you that you want to be for our child?

_____

_____

What are things you do *not* want to bring into your parenting?

_____

_____

How will our different experiences of family life affect what we do as parents?

_____

_____

TO PONDER

Do I have lingering issues, or even trauma, from my childhood that need addressing? How can I get support for this? Do I have concerns about my partner's ability to be the kind of parent we want for our baby? How can I show compassion for and support my partner toward healing and growth?

A MOMENT FOR ME
"Inner Child" Exploration

The profound connection between mother and baby is deepened as you start to connect with and attach to your own inner child. The gift of motherhood is an opportunity to get to know yourself in a deeper, more authentic and childlike way. Many moms describe the journey as spiritual. The beautiful innocence of your childhood gets blurry as life happens, but what if you could momentarily return to that innocence and connect with your inner child? This alternating nostril breath practice helps connect the right and left sides of the brain. As you inhale, think about the pure and childlike place in your heart, and as you exhale, send that pure love to each part of you. This can be practiced anytime and anywhere, but try to choose a place in the house that allows for peace.

1 Close your eyes and connect with your heart and breath as you feel your chest rising and falling.

2 Using your dominant hand, place the forefinger between your eyebrows (this helps calm the nervous system and represents intuition), the thumb on one nostril, and the pinky on the other.

3 Using your thumb, close the nostril and inhale. Then, using the pinky, close the other nostril (so both nostrils are closed), hold the breath for a moment, lift the thumb, and exhale. Repeat this cycle for a few minutes.

Self-Care Check In

On a scale of 1 to 10, where 1 means "really struggling" and 10 means "no problem":

What is my current stress level?

1 2 3 4 5 6 7 8 9 10

What is my current level of joy?

1 2 3 4 5 6 7 8 9 10

How am I doing on my self-talk/thought life?

1 2 3 4 5 6 7 8 9 10

Am I making nutrition and hydration a priority?

1 2 3 4 5 6 7 8 9 10

Am I managing my mental health?

1 2 3 4 5 6 7 8 9 10

Am I getting enough sleep and rest?

1 2 3 4 5 6 7 8 9 10

How am I doing at staying present?

1 2 3 4 5 6 7 8 9 10

Am I being supported in my mothering?

1 2 3 4 5 6 7 8 9 10

Am I making enough space for myself and my needs?

1 2 3 4 5 6 7 8 9 10

NOURISHMENT TIP
Hydration

It goes without saying that hydration is vital to your health (especially if you are breastfeeding), but water can get boring. The smoothie recipe below is filled with some of the most hydrating foods. Here are some other ways to stay hydrated:

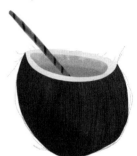

- Add frozen fruit, such as berries, to your water

- Enjoy coconut water

- Try sparkling water with lime

- Slice and enjoy whole, water-rich foods like watermelon, grapes, tomatoes, and celery

- Freeze your smoothie for two hours (it becomes a great ice cream substitute)

- Create a habit of hydrating each time you feed Baby

Hydrating Super-Smoothie

1 small cucumber
1 cup pineapple
1 cup spinach
1 inch fresh ginger root (or 1
   teaspoon dry, ground ginger)
½ cup orange juice
1 cup pure unsweetened coconut water
2 servings plant-based protein powder (such
   as rice, pea, hemp, soy, or a combination)
1 cup Greek yogurt, or kefir
   Cinnamon to taste
1 cup ice

Blend all ingredients in a high-speed
blender. Adjust ingredients to taste.

Serves 2

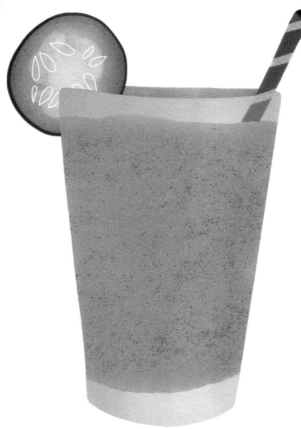

YOUR DEVELOPING PARENTING STYLE

Whether or not you realize it, these early months with your baby can set the tone for the kind of mother you will be. It's important to be mindful of your parenting style, which probably started developing during your pregnancy. Over time, with patient exploration, you will see your parenting style take shape, yet even in the early months you will see clues as to the temperament of your baby, which will affect how you parent.

In order to more authentically inhabit your unique role, you may need to let go of unrealistic expectations and romanticized images. For example, maybe your baby is a very light sleeper or needs more physical connection than you envisioned. Perhaps unexpected challenges have led you to adjust your parenting game plan. Returning to an "I'm doing the best I can with the knowledge I have" mindset can help quell your fears and create space for your own parenting style to flourish.

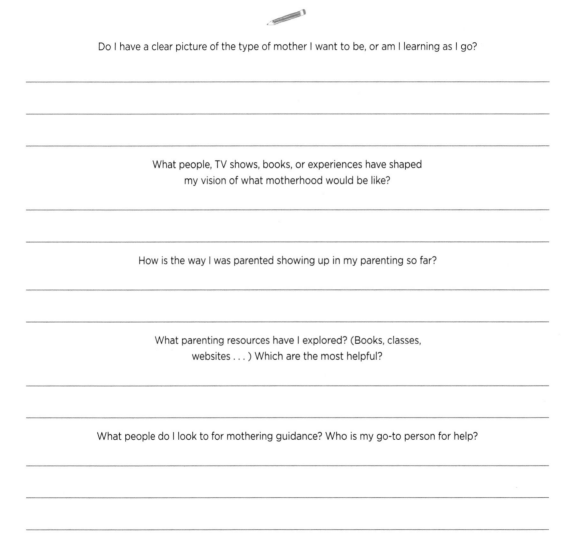

Do I have a clear picture of the type of mother I want to be, or am I learning as I go?

_____

_____

_____

What people, TV shows, books, or experiences have shaped
my vision of what motherhood would be like?

_____

_____

How is the way I was parented showing up in my parenting so far?

_____

_____

What parenting resources have I explored? (Books, classes,
websites . . .) Which are the most helpful?

_____

_____

What people do I look to for mothering guidance? Who is my go-to person for help?

_____

_____

_____

How does social media shape me as a mother?

_____

_____

_____

What did I *swear* I would never do before Baby arrived that I am now doing?

_____

_____

How would I describe Baby's temperament, and what does
that bring out in me as a woman and a mom?

_____

_____

_____

_____

TO PONDER

Are there parenting styles that I see around me
that I find myself judging or criticizing?
Have I been judged for my parenting choices? How have I navigated that?

A MOMENT FOR ME
Reflections of a First-time Mom

"I've wanted to be a mom for as long as I can remember. I've had this vision in my head and heart of what being a mom looks and feels like. Well, what I've learned so far is that my reality now far surpasses anything I could have envisioned, in both the joyful and the painful things. I had a mental block about how my husband would read my mind and always help without being asked. I thought I would suddenly have total contentment and my life's meaning would be complete. What I have experienced instead is a more authentic version of my dreams played out in the real world. As I let go of my preconceived ideas and show up each day with a clean slate, I see there is more room for my own parenting style to develop." (Erin Sears Basile, first-time mom)

NAVIGATING DIFFICULT CHOICES

Whether your experience so far has been smooth sailing or the opposite, there often seem to be difficult situations to navigate and decisions to make. No matter how much you have prepared yourself, some decisions can feel overwhelming, even paralyzing, especially in early motherhood. From decisions about medical care to sleep arrangements, from budgeting to parenting choices, being a parent can seem synonymous with making hard choices. What can feel so overwhelming is the fear of the unknown, and fear is what robs us of peace and joy. Take some deep breaths and have confidence that you will do what you feel is best for your baby at the time, and give yourself grace if you need to adjust your choices. The path will become clearer as you walk it one step at a time.

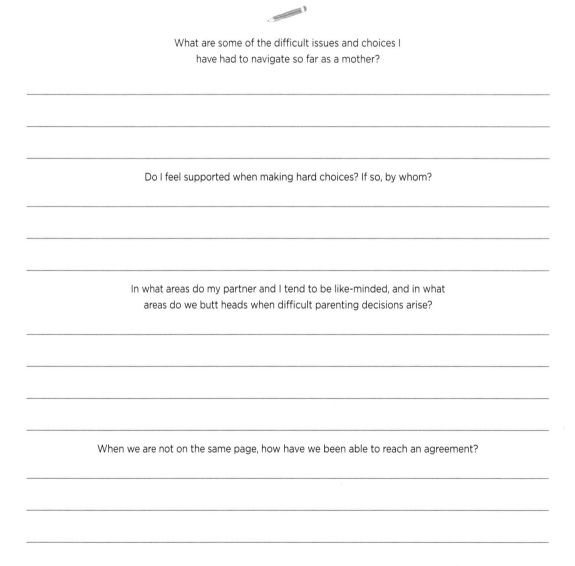

What are some of the difficult issues and choices I
have had to navigate so far as a mother?

_____

_____

_____

Do I feel supported when making hard choices? If so, by whom?

_____

_____

_____

In what areas do my partner and I tend to be like-minded, and in what
areas do we butt heads when difficult parenting decisions arise?

_____

_____

_____

_____

When we are not on the same page, how have we been able to reach an agreement?

_____

_____

_____

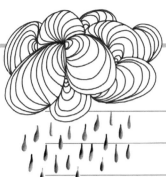

What decisions are looming and will need to be addressed?

_____

_____

_____

_____

_____

What decisions need to be addressed now, and what can wait?

_____

_____

_____

_____

_____

TO PONDER

What feelings come up for me when an important decision is looming?
What has navigating difficult choices taught me about myself?

A MOMENT FOR ME
How Important Is It?

Navigating difficult decisions can seem overwhelming, especially if you and your partner aren't on the same page. Many things may feel out of your control; however, you *are* in control of how you approach and react to things. Consider these suggestions the next time you are making a difficult decision that might lead to conflict.

Choose a calm space and time of
   day to address things.
Choose an activity that you both enjoy, like
   hiking, and talk while you walk.
Stay grounded and trust your intuition.

Wrap yourself and your partner with compassion
   like a gentle blanket. Remember that
   things may seem extra heavy when fear,
   lack of sleep, and stress are factors.
Take one thing at a time. Perhaps you don't
   have to plan out the next eighteen
   years of Baby's life in one sitting.
Share with your partner through
   the lens of love, not fear.
If you have a spiritual practice, then pray, and trust.
Place your wants, needs, fears, and desires into
   a "God box" or "universe box" as an exercise
   in giving your feelings and concerns over to
   something more powerful than yourself.

Final Reflections

In the commitment of each to the other in the marriage,
the two pseudo-selfs fuse into a new emotional oneness.

MURRAY BOWEN

With the unity of my marriage at the forefront of my mind,
what are my reflections on growing my emotional oneness
with myself, and then between me and my partner?

_____

_____

_____

_____

_____

What did becoming a mother teach me or show me about myself
recently? How can I carry this lesson throughout my life?

_____

_____

_____

What have I read, watched, or listened to recently that I want to remember?

_____

_____

_____

What worries or fears about motherhood have I been able to work through?

_____

_____

_____

What thoughts can I be mindful of that decrease my joy and peace, and
how can I best work through them and, if needed, get support?

_____

_____

_____

_____

How have I surprised myself or made myself proud as a mother?

_____

_____

_____

What do I want to let go of that is not serving me well?

_____

_____

_____

What would my future self want to say to me right now?

_____

_____

_____

A commitment, declaration, intention, or promise to myself moving forward
that helps me hold tight to what I have learned in this chapter:

_____

_____

_____

_____

_____

A Love Note to Myself

Take some time to truly appreciate all that you are and all that you do for yourself, your baby, and those around you. Celebrate YOU in writing and memorialize the parts of yourself that deserve love and acknowledgment. Return to your words from time to time when you need a reminder.

Dear Me,

_____

_____

_____

_____

_____

_____

_____

_____

_____

_____

_____

_____

_____

_____

_____

Draw, doodle, or attach pictures that describe
the essence of you becoming a mother.

6

YOUR COMMUNITY

Much of your motherhood experience will be shaped by those around you—your immediate and extended families, friends, and the new community of mothers you may feel drawn to be part of. How much you'll experience this pull depends on your personality and unique situation—some mothers may feel ready early on to join new-mom groups, while others may want to stay cocooned with Baby. This special, fleeting time in your life highlights the dichotomy between wanting to continue to hibernate with Baby and the longing for connection. It's important to honor both feelings in your own time. Simply knowing that other moms are out there going though similar triumphs and challenges can be reassuring in and of itself, but the time will present itself when you are ready to expand your tribe. This—new friends who understand the struggles and joys of parenthood—can be a nourishing and valuable perk of your new life stage.

For many moms, having a new baby brings the desire to create stronger ties with extended family. Family are often our biggest source of support and celebration, yet there may be some challenges to navigate. And while your tribe may consist mainly of family members, you will likely also begin to find close friends who end up becoming like family. Allow your family and friend community to hold you up, and continue to lean toward those who bring positivity, authenticity, and joy into your life.

Comparison and loneliness are two pitfalls many moms must watch out for. They are often felt most in the early years of motherhood, and they have the potential to cloud the beauty of this time and bring further disconnection down the road. Practicing balance and compassion when comparison and loneliness creep in is a gentle ebb and flow. By journaling, you can work through these feelings, and all the complexities that come with them, to help you live this beautiful time in a whole, authentic way.

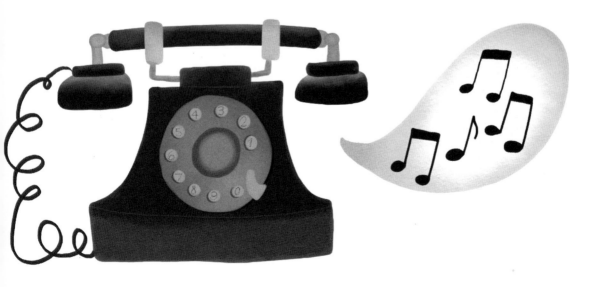

I believe we do all have the biological hardwiring for a parenting instinct, and this instinct comes through in flying colors when we feel well supported and nurtured by our families and communities.

ROBIN GRILLE, PSYCHOLOGIST

What does my community look like and in what ways has my community supported and nurtured my parenting instinct?

_____

_____

_____

_____

_____

_____

_____

_____

_____

_____

_____

_____

_____

_____

_____

_____

_____

_____

_____

_____

MY PEOPLE

Maybe you too have found that becoming a mom simultaneously shrinks and expands your social circle. During the first few months with Baby, those you consider "your people" hopefully showed up big time. Those precious visitors who helped welcome Baby into the world, who served you meals and supported you with a helping hand, listening ear, and shoulder to cry on are treasures. And there is a sweet spot after Baby arrives in which you may want to stay in the safety and comfort of your nest with "your people." Yet there comes a time when you want to open up socially and relationally as you crave more adult contact. You may want to expand your tribe to include other moms in your same life stage—especially if not many of those in your circle have babies. The song that goes, "Make new friends, but keep the old, one is silver and the other gold" resonates in the life of a mom.

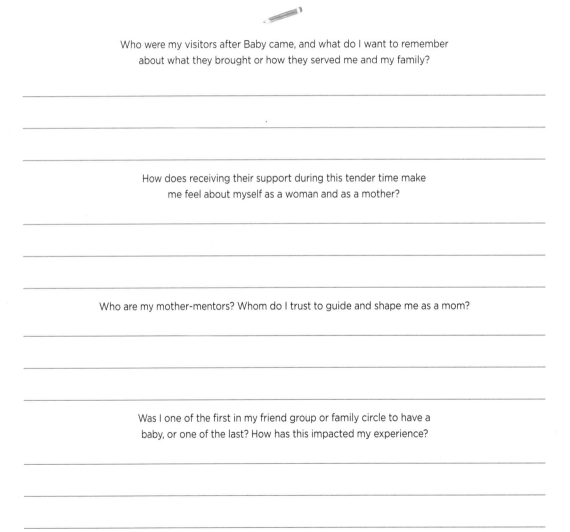

Who were my visitors after Baby came, and what do I want to remember
about what they brought or how they served me and my family?

_____

_____

_____

How does receiving their support during this tender time make
me feel about myself as a woman and as a mother?

_____

_____

_____

Who are my mother-mentors? Whom do I trust to guide and shape me as a mom?

_____

_____

_____

Was I one of the first in my friend group or family circle to have a
baby, or one of the last? How has this impacted my experience?

_____

_____

_____

What are some funny, unexpected, or cute things my friends
have said as they experience me being a mom?

_____

_____

In what ways have my closest friendships shifted since Baby came?

_____

_____

Whom would I consider to be my tribe, or whom would I like to have in my
tribe? Whom would I consider to be my closest confidant, the person I can share
anything with? Or, is there someone I have a hunch might become that person?

_____

_____

_____

What mom groups or activities do I resonate with the best? What drains my energy?

_____

_____

TO PONDER

Do I feel disconnected from my friends who don't have
kids? In what ways can I keep those connections?
Has anyone close to me said or done something that has
hurt me or caused a rift? How have I navigated that?

A MOMENT FOR ME
Mommy-Group Multitasking

Consider trying moms groups like mommy-and-me yoga, walking groups, and stroller fitness classes. This way you can combine many self-care needs, like getting out of the house, exercising, and meeting like-minded moms. Beware energy drains or negative attitudes. Your time and emotional energy are very precious, so be sure to invest only in relationships and activities that edify you and help you feel like your best self.

LONELINESS

Many moms with young babies spend their days alone and on their own. This in itself is not a problem—in your time alone with Baby you are establishing a rhythm and creating lasting bonds. Yet there is a point where *being* alone can turn into *feeling* alone, which can easily turn into loneliness. Feeling left out, disconnected, and isolated can easily turn into feeling resentful, full of blame, and even depressed. All of this is common, especially during the early years of motherhood, though it requires care and attention to keep these complex feelings from hindering this joyful and exciting time of life. Confide in a close friend or even seek help from a professional if these feelings become unmanageable, especially if feelings of loneliness still come up often regardless of how much support is available.

In what circumstances during this new season do I
most feel disconnected or left out?

How frequently does my sense of disconnection turn into loneliness?

How can I work through these feelings or shift the
situation so that resentment does not set in?

Am I getting stuck in blaming mode? If so, who takes the
brunt of it? (Baby, my partner, myself . . .)

How does my self-talk play a role in my feelings of isolation or loneliness?

_____

_____

_____

What are some unhelpful things I do when I feel alone or resentful? (Eat junk food, wallow, numb out, blame, have a pity party, escape to social media . . .)

_____

_____

_____

What are some activities that can help me shift my mindset? (Call a friend, sing, exercise, pray, meditate, nap, find something productive to do . . .)

_____

_____

_____

TO PONDER

Do I recognize being alone with Baby as a natural part of this
life stage? Or are feelings of loneliness becoming overwhelming,
veering toward what some new moms describe as "crazy"?
What role did loneliness play in my life before I became a mom?

A MOMENT FOR ME
Mommy Mantra, "I Am Not Alone"

I know I am not alone, even if it may feel that way in this moment. My feelings are not facts. As I allow myself to feel, I allow myself to heal. I connect with mamas all over the world who feel lonely at times. I see them, and they see me. I honor my feelings by stepping out of my comfort zone and getting support. I draw near to women and family who will lift me up. I honor the growing pains and welcome new connections.

Self-Care Check In

On a scale of 1 to 10, where 1 means "really struggling" and 10 means "no problem":

What is my current stress level?

1   2   3   4   5   6   7   8   9   10

What is my current level of joy?

1   2   3   4   5   6   7   8   9   10

How am I doing on my self-talk/thought life?

1   2   3   4   5   6   7   8   9   10

Am I making nutrition and hydration a priority?

1   2   3   4   5   6   7   8   9   10

Am I managing my mental health?

1   2   3   4   5   6   7   8   9   10

Am I getting enough sleep and rest?

1   2   3   4   5   6   7   8   9   10

How am I doing at staying present?

1   2   3   4   5   6   7   8   9   10

Am I being supported in my mothering?

1   2   3   4   5   6   7   8   9   10

Am I making enough space for myself and my needs?

1   2   3   4   5   6   7   8   9   10

NOURISHMENT TIP
Protein Power

The word "protein" comes from the Greek *protos*, meaning "first." This nutrient is the basic element of living cells, of first importance. Protein is the building block of the human body, and we need a steady supply of it to build and repair organs, muscles, antibodies, hormones, and enzymes—every single component of the body. Aim for at least half a gram of protein per pound of body weight. So, a 150-pound woman should aim for about 75 grams each day. Good sources of protein include eggs, tofu, seafood, lean meats, beans, nuts, seeds, and dairy.

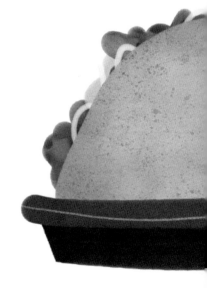

Simple Salsa Verde Chicken with Beans

You can add this tasty chicken filling to corn or wheat tortillas, salads, or burrito bowls.

  1 pound organic, free-range, skinless
      and boneless chicken breasts
  ½ cup salsa verde
  1 cup shredded green cabbage
  ¼ cup chopped onion
  1 can pinto or black beans

Combine the chicken and salsa in a slow cooker. Cook on low for 6 hours or on high for 4 hours.

You can also simmer on the stove on low heat in a covered pot until fully cooked.

Add the beans for the last hour.

Before serving, shred the chicken with a fork and sprinkle cabbage and onion on top as desired.

Double the recipe and freeze half!

Serves 4

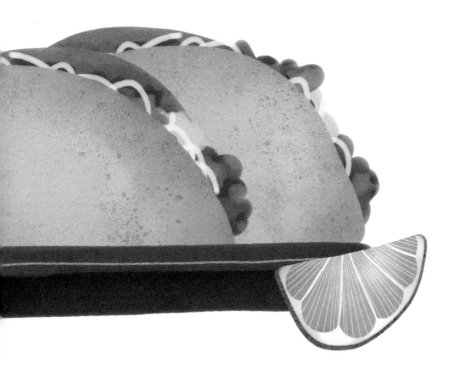

COMPARISON

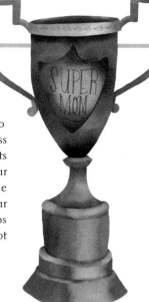

One of the downsides of being part of a community, especially where motherhood is concerned, is the tendency to compare oneself to others. While observing those around you and getting tips on social media can add value to your life, it becomes unhealthy when you wind up feeling less confident in yourself, or more self-critical, as a result. Comparing yourself to others can be a subtle behavior pattern, and seemingly harmless, but it has the potential to steal your joy and breed discontentment. When you're busy being critical of yourself, you vastly diminish the value of your own experience. Many moms find that their striving to be the "perfect" mom makes it difficult to enjoy being a mom. Don't miss all the little magical moments and mom wins that make up your day. Take time to appreciate the gifts and talents you bring to your motherhood journey. It helps to remember: your baby is not making comparisons.

In what ways do I compare my situation with that of other mothers?

_____

_____

Where do I find these comparisons lead me?

_____

_____

In what ways do I think others compare themselves, either in a negative or positive way, to me and my situation? What kind of perspective does this bring?

_____

_____

In what ways am I content with who I am and where I'm at? Who or what contributes to my contentment?

_____

_____

In what ways am I discontent with who I am and where I'm at? Who or what contributes to my discontentment?

_____

_____

How does social media play a role in that?

_____

_____

In what ways, consciously or subconsciously, do I expect myself to be the "perfect mother"? Do I perceive those around me as having unrealistic expectations of me?

_____

_____

In what ways can I shift any unrealistic expectations I have for myself, and how can I extend more grace and compassion to myself?

_____

_____

TO PONDER

Have I struggled with comparison in earlier parts of my life? How can I leverage my new role as a mom to break any comparison or perfectionism tendencies?

A MOMENT FOR ME
The Comparison Struggle

Where your thoughts go, your energy will follow. Turn your thoughts toward the amazing blessing it is to be a mom exactly the way YOU do it. When comparison sneaks in to steal your joy, remember that you have everything you need inside of you, and allow comparison to become acceptance through the following practice. Visceral, physical acceptance of the moment helps foster mental and emotional acceptance.

LEGS-UP-THE-WALL POSE
Lie on your bed or the floor with your legs propped up on the headboard or wall (so your body forms an L shape). A pillow might feel nice under your hips. Your hands can either relax to the sides of your body (palms facing up), or rest one hand on your belly and one hand on your heart. Keep your legs straight up and about hip-width distance apart, and begin to allow gravity to release the muscle fibers starting with your feet and continuing through each muscle group until you arrive at the top of your head. Use a slow, steady breath, inhaling and exhaling to the count of four, to connect within. With each breath, allow a positive attribute to be your focus, such as, "I am loving, I am capable, I am unique, I am enough." By honoring exactly where you are, you begin to loosen the discontentment that can lead to comparison. This is also very calming to the nervous system and allows the mind-body connection to grow.

EXTENDED-FAMILY CHALLENGES

Family is an integral part of your tribe/community. Since it's common nowadays for families to be scattered, distance can often keep you from having the kind of connection you desire. It can be disappointing not to have certain family members there with you, experiencing this golden time in your life and bonding with your baby. While things like FaceTime and social media can help, the distance is still felt on both sides. On the other hand, you may have local family who have become emotionally distant because of differing lifestyles. Now that you have a baby, you have a compelling reason to reconnect—a new baby has the beautiful potential to bring people back together. Perhaps this is the time to let go of whatever was keeping you apart. That said, there may be family members who have strong views on parenting that don't align with yours, or perhaps you have a large family with big personalities and energy. Too much of a good thing can disrupt the harmony of your new family unit, so finding balance in this area is key.

With whom in my extended family do I feel connected, and what keeps us connected?

_____

_____

_____

_____

Whom do I feel disconnected from, and how did that come about?
(Living far away, personality, differences . . .)

_____

_____

_____

In what creative ways can Baby and I stay connected
with family who do not live local to us?

_____

_____

_____

_____

In what ways do my family support me as a woman and as a mother?

_____

_____

If there has been a relationship with family (or friends) that has suffered
because of differing opinions about parenting, how have I handled it?

_____

_____

Do I have unrealistic expectations of family members?
How can I bring that into balance?

_____

_____

_____

TO PONDER

What relationships, if any, need boundaries to keep the
relationship mutually healthy, and what does that look like?
Are there any past traumas or struggles with family that need
to be addressed or healed that I am responsible for?

A MOMENT FOR ME
Rewards (Other than Food) for Making it Through a Challenging Week

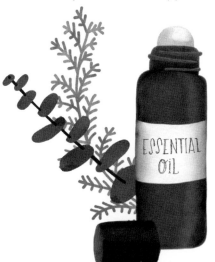

Get a pedicure
Give yourself an Epsom salts foot
   soak with essential oils
Take a shower that lasts longer than three minutes
Buy a new pair of cute shoes
Get yourself an outfit that makes you
   feel like the beauty you are
Watch a movie from your bucket list
Take a yoga class
Buy your favorite flowers

Final Reflections

It will help us and our children if we can laugh at our faults. It will help us tolerate our shortcomings, and it will help our children see that the goal is to be a human, not perfect.

RABBI NEIL KURSHAN

After exploring the roles comparison and loneliness play in my life,
how can this guide me to a new level of self-acceptance?

_____

_____

_____

_____

What did becoming a mother teach me or show me about myself
recently? How can I carry this lesson throughout my life?

_____

_____

_____

_____

What have I read, watched, or listened to recently that I want to remember?

_____

_____

_____

What worries or fears about motherhood have I been able to work through?

_____

_____

_____

_____

What thoughts can I be mindful of that decrease my joy and peace, and
how can I best work through them and, if needed, get support?

_____

_____

_____

How have I surprised myself or made myself proud as a mother?

_____

_____

What do I want to let go of that is not serving me well?

_____

_____

What would my future self want to say to me right now?

_____

_____

A commitment, declaration, intention, or promise to myself moving forward
that helps me hold tight to what I have learned in this chapter:

_____

_____

_____

_____

A Love Note to Myself

Take some time to truly appreciate all that you are and all that you do for yourself, your baby, and those around you. Celebrate YOU in writing and memorialize the parts of yourself that deserve love and acknowledgment. Return to your words from time to time when you need a reminder.

Dear Me,

_____

_____

_____

_____

_____

_____

_____

_____

_____

_____

_____

_____

_____

_____

_____

Draw, doodle, or attach pictures that describe
the essence of you becoming a mother.

7
MY RELATIONSHIP
WITH MY BABY

By now you have likely come to know that the mother-baby connection is truly unlike any other relationship in the world. And it's one that will grow and change along with you and your baby. This connection helps shape you as a mother, in both how you care for and communicate with Baby, and guides your mother's intuition. It is well worth intentionally investing in this connection—it can serve as an anchor when challenges arise and will be a foundation of trust for the future.

The intimate bond that you are forming will allow you to see from your child's perspective, to help assess what Baby needs. When you are connected and in tune with your baby, you will grow to trust this beautiful little teacher looking back at you as you learn to translate Baby's cues. What a special dance of love, compassion, and openness to take part in together!

No advice from books, doctors, family members, or friends can take the place of your mother's intuition. *You* are the expert on your baby. Yet the sad reality is that a mother's intuition can be threatened by all of the differing views on sensitive subjects. Part of your role as a mom is finding a balance between trusting what you know is right for you and your baby and being open to guidance from those around you. There are some parenting choices that are very personal and complex and that call for exploration on your own terms. This can spark insecurity and fear, but it is also a chance for layers of you to evolve. Allow patience and love to carry you through these raw and vulnerable moments when your resolve is tested, knowing that the two of you will find your way together.

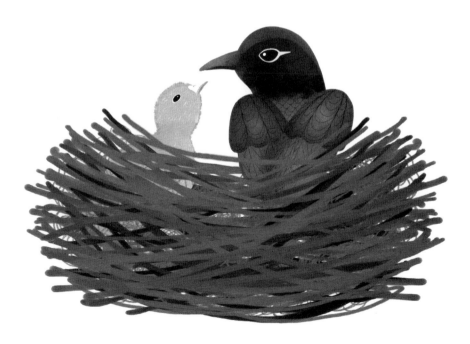

Inside, you give your body and your blood; outside, you give your milk, your eyes, your hands, your voice — your entire self. Your baby gazes intently at you, studying your face as if to say, 'I know already that you are the most important person in my world.'

WILLIAM SEARS

As I dive deeper into my relationship with Baby and my intuition grows, what excites me about this phase of motherhood? What is challenging me?

YOUR INTUITION

A mother's intuition is grounded in information collected by all of her senses. It is a feature of motherhood that allows a mother keen and quick insight into the needs of her baby, usually independent of reasoning. This intuition is something that is often talked about, but it does not truly become clear until you experience it. And more clarity comes as you practice listening to the "gut feeling" that is there to guide you. It is an innate knowing that grows and develops and will continue to serve you throughout your motherhood journey. You may find yourself saying, "I just know." And it's true: no one knows your child better than you do. You may receive well-meaning criticism for some of your choices from people who have different opinions on child raising, but don't let that deter you from leaning into what your mother's intuition tells you. Your intuition is nature's way of protecting your baby and ensuring your baby's needs are met.

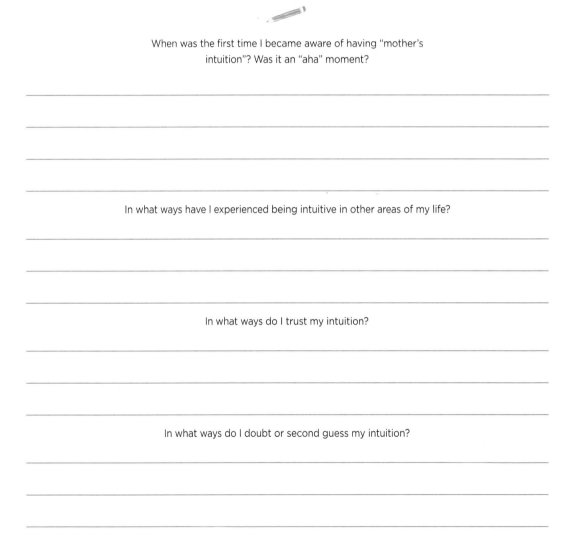

When was the first time I became aware of having "mother's intuition"? Was it an "aha" moment?

_____

_____

_____

_____

In what ways have I experienced being intuitive in other areas of my life?

_____

_____

In what ways do I trust my intuition?

_____

_____

In what ways do I doubt or second guess my intuition?

_____

_____

Who are the people in my life who encourage tapping into my mother's intuition?

_____

_____

_____

Are there certain things or people that hinder or block my inner voice from being heard
or recognized? How can I clear a path for my intuition to flourish unencumbered?

_____

_____

_____

_____

_____

TO PONDER

How has my mother's intuition enhanced my experience of motherhood?
How do I envision my new intuition guiding my motherhood long term?
What has my intuition taught me about myself as a woman?

A MOMENT FOR ME
Trust Affirmation

Today I will embrace all that I am.
I trust my feelings and insights as a mother.
Today I am completely in tune with my
   inner wisdom and my baby's needs.
I am filled with a mother's light
   of love, peace, and joy.

Today I see each moment as a fresh opportunity
   to express my fullness and value as a mom.
My mother's intuition leads me
   to the right decisions.
Where peace dwells, fear cannot.
I am exactly where I am supposed to be today.

YOUR BABY'S CUES

Many new mothers wonder how they will know what their baby needs. While there are plenty of resources available to help with this, and plenty of people to advise you, your baby will usually be your best guide. If your baby is hungry, tired, cold or hot, scared, in pain, over-stimulated or simply needs to be held, your baby will let you know. Your baby's cries are her language and the primary way she communicates with you. Over time you will learn to distinguish what each kind of cry means. Usually, though, babies start giving clues and cues about their needs well before they get to the crying stage. The value of being in tune with Baby and intentionally exploring this often subtle communication is that you can usually meet a need even before Baby has to cry for it. The more you practice being responsive, the more you will trust your baby's cues to guide you. And as you respond to them, your baby will come to trust that you are listening.

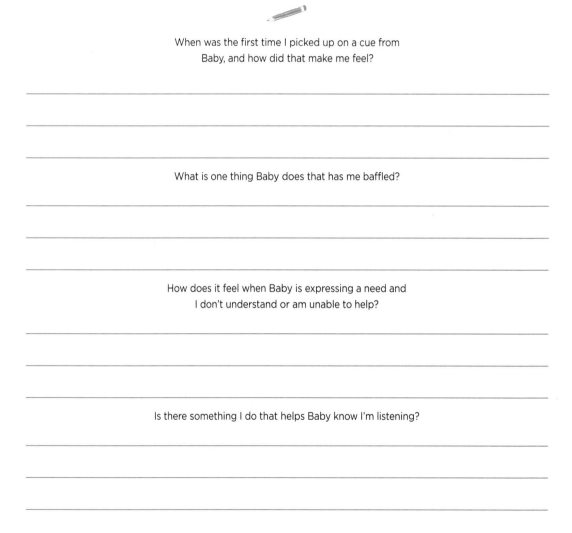

When was the first time I picked up on a cue from
Baby, and how did that make me feel?

_____

_____

_____

What is one thing Baby does that has me baffled?

_____

_____

_____

How does it feel when Baby is expressing a need and
I don't understand or am unable to help?

_____

_____

_____

Is there something I do that helps Baby know I'm listening?

_____

_____

_____

What resources or forms of guidance have been
helpful to me in translating Baby's cues?

_____

_____

_____

What is something Baby does that validates my response, as
if to say, "Yay, Mom, you got it!"? How does that feel?

_____

_____

_____

How have I grown in my ability to recognize and respond to Baby's cues?

_____

_____

_____

TO PONDER

What is it like to know that my baby and I have
a "secret language" that is unique to us?
Are there times when my mother's intuition scares me?

A MOMENT FOR ME
Laugh!

They say that a child laughs an average of 300 times each day, but an adult only laughs five times. Don't let Baby be the only one to receive the myriad benefits of laughter!

What makes you laugh? Here are some ways to laugh more often:

Listen to a silly podcast or watch a funny movie
Have a lighthearted conversation with friends
    and family who have a funny bone
Laugh at yourself when you have a
    mommy-brain moment
Have a girl's night out to the latest comedy
    blockbuster or comedy club

Self-Care Check In

On a scale of 1 to 10, where 1 means "really struggling" and 10 means "no problem":

What is my current stress level?

1   2   3   4   5   6   7   8   9   10

What is my current level of joy?

1   2   3   4   5   6   7   8   9   10

How am I doing on my self-talk/thought life?

1   2   3   4   5   6   7   8   9   10

Am I making nutrition and hydration a priority?

1   2   3   4   5   6   7   8   9   10

Am I managing my mental health?

1   2   3   4   5   6   7   8   9   10

Am I getting enough sleep and rest?

1   2   3   4   5   6   7   8   9   10

How am I doing at staying present?

1   2   3   4   5   6   7   8   9   10

Am I being supported in my mothering?

1   2   3   4   5   6   7   8   9   10

Am I making enough space for myself and my needs?

1   2   3   4   5   6   7   8   9   10

NOURISHMENT TIP
Healthy Fats

Most Americans eat an excess amount of unhealthy fats (especially animal and hydrogenated fats) and not enough healthy fat (from plants and seafood). Remember that your brain is 60% fat, so we need fat to function properly. Fats also act as a sponge for absorbing fat-soluble vitamins like A, K, D, and E. Healthy fats, like the ones in the recipe and the list below, help regulate immune function and blood pressure, protect organs from injury, and keep our moods stable. It's helpful to keep in mind that we need a "right-fat diet," not a "low-fat diet." For more information about healthy fats, see our recommended resources in the back of the book.

Top healthy fats:

- Pumpkin and sunflower seeds
- Wild salmon
- Walnuts
- Olives
- Nut butters
- Flaxseeds
- Chia seeds
- Avocado

Chocolate-Avocado Pudding

    1 large avocado, peeled and sliced
    1 ripe banana
1½ teaspoons vanilla extract
    ¼ cup unsweetened cocoa powder
    1 serving chocolate plant-based
       protein powder (optional)
    ¼ cup full-fat canned coconut milk
       Pinch cinnamon
       Chocolate chips to taste

Place all ingredients (except the chocolate chips) in a food processor or blender and pulse for 1 to 2 minutes, or until desired texture.

Chill for 30 minutes if desired.

Top with chocolate chips before serving.

Serves 2

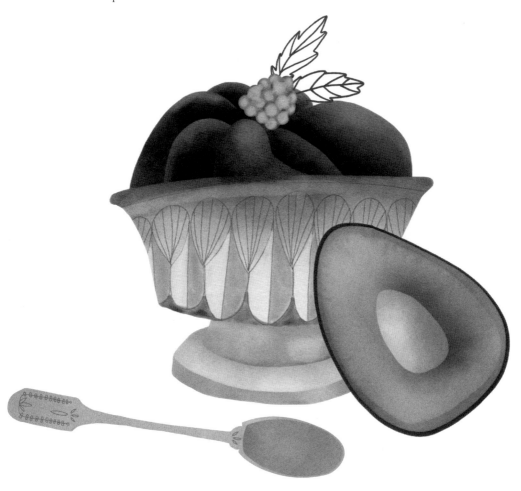

COMMUNICATION

Verbal and nonverbal communication are the main ways we connect. The words we use, and particularly the ways we use them, have power. By understanding our tone, inflection, and facial expressions, those around us interpret our words. This is especially true for babies who don't yet have spoken language. Babies understand our inflection and tone before they understand our words—even when we are talking aloud to ourselves. Whether you realize it or not, through how you speak, you are teaching your baby communication patterns—so it's a good idea to attend to tone and inflection and the emotions behind them. Keeping in mind that managing your emotions will likely be a lifelong process, this is a perfect time to practice. Sometimes simply taking some deep breaths or a pause before speaking will help your tone of voice be what you want to model to Baby. When communication is done with patience, compassion, and mindfulness, there is more space for beautiful two-way communication to develop and flourish.

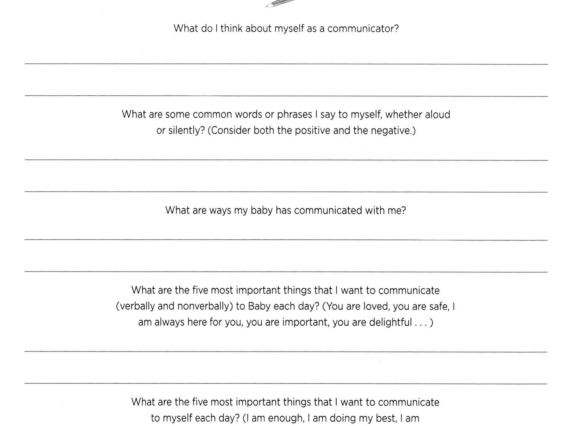

What do I think about myself as a communicator?

_____

_____

What are some common words or phrases I say to myself, whether aloud
or silently? (Consider both the positive and the negative.)

_____

_____

What are ways my baby has communicated with me?

_____

_____

What are the five most important things that I want to communicate
(verbally and nonverbally) to Baby each day? (You are loved, you are safe, I
am always here for you, you are important, you are delightful . . .)

_____

_____

What are the five most important things that I want to communicate
to myself each day? (I am enough, I am doing my best, I am
cherished, I am beautiful, I can do hard things, I am worthy . . .)

_____

_____

Am I aware of my negative nonverbal communication? What am I
most frequently communicating, and how does that look? (Anxious
or stressful energy, tension in the body, shallow breathing . . .)

_____

_____

_____

TO PONDER

Do I notice how I communicate with myself spilling
over into how I communicate with Baby?
Do I have unhealthy communication patterns from the past
that need attention, and how can I get support for this?

A MOMENT FOR ME
Negative Self-talk Makeover

The constant mental work it takes to be a mom can easily lead to mommy guilt and mommy burnout. Becoming more mindful of your inner dialogue and thought patterns is the first step toward moving them from negative to inspiring. Here are common thought patterns many moms experience and ideas for how to reframe those thoughts away from your "negative inner critic" to your "inspirational inner angel."

NEGATIVE INNER CRITIC	INSPIRATIONAL INNER ANGEL
"Self-care is selfish; I don't have time."	"I honor my body so I can be a healthy, connected mama and set an example for my kids."
"I am not good enough."	"I am in the midst of a precious time in my baby's life. 'Good enough' is good enough!"
"My partner isn't attracted to me."	"My body created a life and my partner has a new appreciation for its beauty."
"I am a bad mom for having to go back to work."	"I am providing for my family's needs and showing my kids that they can be whoever they want to be."
"I have no idea what I'm doing."	"I trust my intuition and it's okay to learn as I go."

RITUALS AND PLAY

Rituals, or comforting routines, allow us to move through tasks in a way that brings structure and ease. The mind and body thrive on the rhythms of routine, letting us enjoy the present moment in a state of calm. Rituals can incorporate activities like prayer, singing, reading, mantras/affirmations, infant massage, dance/movement, and playfulness. Many rituals with Baby will involve play, which is one of the main ways your baby will learn. For some moms creating rituals for play may come naturally, but other moms may need to be more intentional. Some moms may even feel like they need to give *themselves* permission to let loose and play with their baby. Being silly and joyful is a beautiful way for Mama and Baby to connect. Take some time to remember the rituals you enjoyed in your childhood. You might also ask your mom what rituals you two enjoyed together when you were a baby.

What rituals have I created around caregiving in the following areas?

Feeding: _____

Diaper changing: _____

Bedtime: _____

Comforting: _____

Bathtime: _____

Car rides: _____

How do these rituals enrich my experience of motherhood?

_____

_____

_____

What kinds of rituals or play am I looking forward
to introducing now and in the future?

_____

_____

_____

_____

What are some things I am teaching Baby through play?

_____

_____

Are there activities I feel like I "should" be doing with Baby that I'm not?

_____

_____

How can I keep playtime with Baby fun and interesting for me?

_____

_____

TO PONDER

Do I struggle with allowing myself to be silly or playful, or does
it come naturally to me? Take some time to explore this.
In what ways have I seen my silly or playful side
come out since becoming a mother?

A MOMENT FOR ME
Peaceful Rituals for Mom

Apply mid-afternoon energizing essential oils (peppermint, citrus). Look for a roller-bottle to apply the oil on your temple, or simply breathe in the aroma.

Relax your shoulders and deepen your breath during Baby's feedings.

Play a calming or uplifting music selection while driving.

Calming breath: Make the exhale longer than the inhale. Inhale for a count of four, exhale for six.

Have a bedtime gratitude prayer/gratitude practice. This is also a very special thing to model for your baby. List five things you are grateful for either out loud or in your thoughts, and attach them to the five senses. Example: "I am grateful that I can see the beautiful fall leaves."

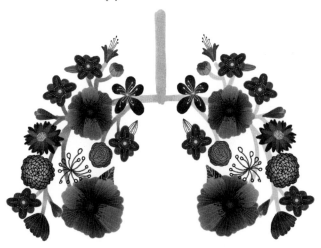

Final Reflections

Listen to the whisper before it becomes a shout.

LORI BREGMAN

How can "listening to the whisper" from my baby and from my own spirit
"before it becomes a shout" enhance my motherhood experience?

_____

_____

_____

_____

What did becoming a mother teach me or show me about myself
recently? How can I carry this lesson throughout my life?

_____

_____

_____

_____

What have I read, watched, or listened to recently that I want to remember?

_____

_____

_____

What worries or fears about motherhood have I been able to work through?

_____

_____

_____

_____

What thoughts can I be mindful of that decrease my joy and peace, and
how can I best work through them and, if needed, get support?

_____

_____

_____

How have I surprised myself or made myself proud as a mother?

_____

_____

What do I want to let go of that is not serving me well?

_____

_____

What would my future self want to say to me right now?

_____

_____

A commitment, declaration, intention, or promise to myself moving forward
that helps me hold tight to what I have learned in this chapter:

_____

_____

_____

A Love Note to Myself

Take some time to truly appreciate all that you are and all that you do for yourself, your baby, and those around you. Celebrate YOU in writing and memorialize the parts of yourself that deserve love and acknowledgment. Return to your words from time to time when you need a reminder.

Dear Me,

_____

_____

_____

_____

_____

_____

_____

_____

_____

_____

_____

_____

_____

_____

Draw, doodle, or attach pictures that describe
the essence of you becoming a mother.

8

MY NEW RHYTHM OF LIFE

"Be ready for your whole world to change," veteran mothers often tell new mothers. Yet the reality this advice entails can only be experienced through living it. The key to withstanding the seismic shift motherhood brings is *balance*. Your balancing act can be graceful, clumsy, unsure, and beautiful, all rolled into one. Just as your baby is exploring and learning new things every day, as a new mother, you are also putting together the puzzle pieces of what your new life with Baby looks like. Some days, you seem to handle everything with grace, in harmony; other days everything falls and crashes like cymbals. The beautiful gift is that each day the rhythm resets and there is a new opportunity to understand and explore. Gradually, what was difficult begins to feel easier. With any new experience comes a learning curve.

One of the tricky things about parenthood is that it demands so much and has the potential to be all-consuming. Yet we must still tend to all the other demands in our life: our household, our work, and our health, which becomes even more important as there is now a precious human relying on us. On top of all that, most new mothers get very little time to do things just for themselves. Be patient with yourself as you practice integrating your previous life's demands into the blessing that is your *new* life's rhythm.

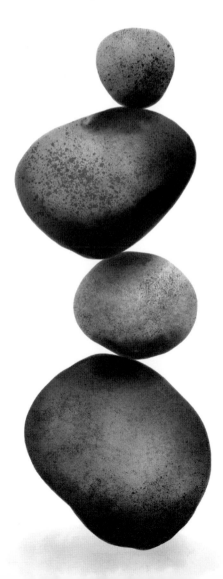

Motherhood brings as much joy as ever, but it still brings
boredom, exhaustion, and sorrow too. Nothing else will
ever make you as happy or as sad, as proud or as tired, for
nothing is quite as hard as helping a person develop his own
individuality — especially while you struggle to keep your own.

MARGUERITE KELLY AND ELIA PARSONS

How do I see myself in this quote?

_____

_____

_____

_____

_____

_____

_____

_____

_____

_____

_____

_____

_____

_____

PLAY AND CREATIVITY!

"If Momma ain't happy, ain't nobody happy!" Truer words have never been spoken. And they highlight why play and creativity need to be a frequent part of a mother's new rhythm of life: it can be so easy for new moms to pour everything into Baby that they forget how to do things simply for the enjoyment of it. Whether because of "mom guilt," lack of motivation, being overly tired or short on time, moms often find a "good" reason to ignore much-needed forms of self-care. Yet those who take time for recreation and self-expression are healthier, happier, more productive, and have more to give their children. The kind of self-care that involves you in recreational activities may look different for you now than before Baby arrived, at least for a while. There is often a natural pruning of the old self to allow our new self to fully blossom, and you may decide that some things that once felt natural no longer fit in your new life. Take some time to recall what brought you joy, excitement, belly laughs, a sense of adventure—and allow your inner child to come out to play and create.

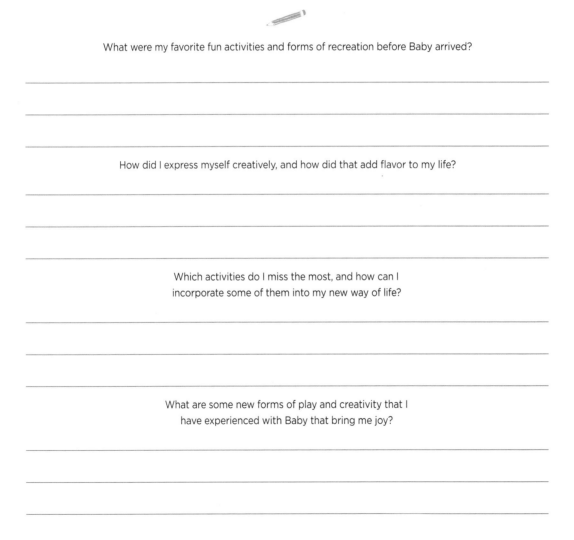

What were my favorite fun activities and forms of recreation before Baby arrived?

_____

_____

_____

How did I express myself creatively, and how did that add flavor to my life?

_____

_____

_____

Which activities do I miss the most, and how can I
incorporate some of them into my new way of life?

_____

_____

_____

What are some new forms of play and creativity that I
have experienced with Baby that bring me joy?

_____

_____

_____

Do I take enough time for play/hobbies/entertainment/
recreation? How can I bring them into balance?

_____

_____

_____

How does taking time for this type of self-care enhance
my experience as a woman and as a mother?

_____

_____

_____

_____

_____

In what ways can I use play and creativity to connect with my partner?

_____

_____

_____

_____

TO PONDER

Are there things I used to do for fun that I feel guilty or resentful
for wanting to still do? Do I resent my partner for having recreation/
creative time? Where might these feelings come from?

A MOMENT FOR ME
Dance Party!

Put on your favorite tunes and dance like no one is watching! Let your "inner child" loose. Watch Baby watching you—notice if he or she reacts differently to you in this state of play. Does it change his or her mood? Babies are little sponges, soaking up and mimicking the sights and sounds around them. Setting a tone that is playful, free, and expressive is a huge gift to you both.

HEALTH HABITS

For many, being a new mom comes with a heightened desire to be healthy physically and nutritionally. This likely started during pregnancy, when you had to eliminate certain unhelpful habits and which may have inspired new, beneficial ones to help grow a healthy baby and support an enjoyable pregnancy. You may have a new awareness now of what you are putting into your mouth and doing with your body that naturally comes with being responsible for a little human. While there are many healthy habits to consider incorporating in your life, pay close attention to the ones that fall into these four areas: food and drink, exercise, sleep, and stress management. Attending to these four areas will greatly impact your energy level, mood, immune system, and overall quality of life. You will soon have even more appreciation for the healthy habits you have created when you see your offspring start to copy them. Modeling this kind of self-respect is an invaluable gift you can offer your family.

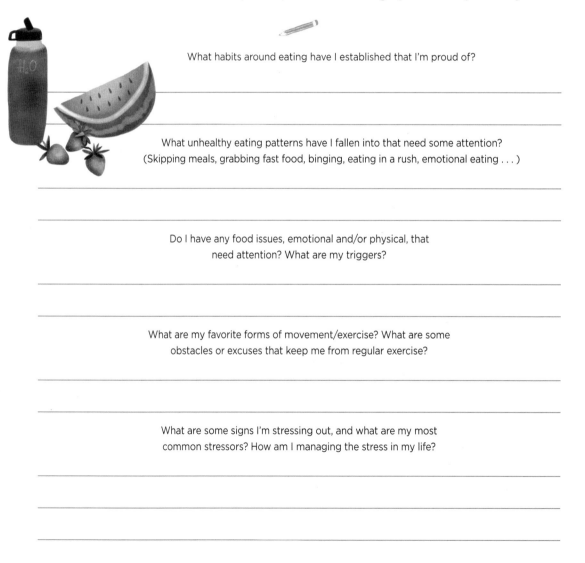

What habits around eating have I established that I'm proud of?

What unhealthy eating patterns have I fallen into that need some attention? (Skipping meals, grabbing fast food, binging, eating in a rush, emotional eating . . .)

Do I have any food issues, emotional and/or physical, that need attention? What are my triggers?

What are my favorite forms of movement/exercise? What are some obstacles or excuses that keep me from regular exercise?

What are some signs I'm stressing out, and what are my most common stressors? How am I managing the stress in my life?

What time-wasters or excuses distract me from paying attention to my health habits?

_____

_____

How have I seen these four main health categories (food and drink, exercise, sleep, and stress management) work together synergistically to establish long-term, stable health?

_____

_____

TO PONDER

Do the people I surround myself with support a healthy
lifestyle, or do I feel like I'm on my own in this?
Do I have a sense of guilt or shame around the topic of long-
term healthy habits? Where does this come from?

A MOMENT FOR ME
Choose This, Not That

You are not alone if you have salty and/or sweet cravings! At the end of a long day, when Baby is in bed, it is very typical for new mothers to decompress with their favorite snack. Or, maybe you have used food in a less-than-healthy way to offset sleep deprivation. Step one, do NOT beat yourself up for this! This mom gig is not easy. Consider these alternatives when the snack attack or sugar-bug hits.

CHOOSE THIS	NOT THAT
Whole-fat Greek yogurt with fresh fruit and honey or coconut-milk ice cream	Ice cream
Air-popped popcorn with olive oil and sea salt	Potato chips
Small piece dark chocolate (see the recipe for Chocolate-Avocado Pudding in chapter 7)	Candy bar
Apple slices spread with nut butter	Packaged baked goods
Rice crackers with cheese or hummus	French fries

Explore other non-food methods of coping, like taking a bath, getting a massage, having a heart-to-heart with a friend, or watching your favorite TV show. Above all else, remember balance. Enjoy your favorite treat on occasion, judgment free!

Self-Care Check In

On a scale of 1 to 10, where 1 means "really struggling" and 10 means "no problem":

What is my current stress level?

1   2   3   4   5   6   7   8   9   10

What is my current level of joy?

1   2   3   4   5   6   7   8   9   10

How am I doing on my self-talk/thought life?

1   2   3   4   5   6   7   8   9   10

Am I making nutrition and hydration a priority?

1   2   3   4   5   6   7   8   9   10

Am I managing my mental health?

1   2   3   4   5   6   7   8   9   10

Am I getting enough sleep and rest?

1   2   3   4   5   6   7   8   9   10

How am I doing at staying present?

1   2   3   4   5   6   7   8   9   10

Am I being supported in my mothering?

1   2   3   4   5   6   7   8   9   10

Am I making enough space for myself and my needs?

1   2   3   4   5   6   7   8   9   10

NOURISHMENT TIP
Omega-3 Fatty Acids

Got "mommy brain"? There's a reason for this: you may be undernourished in terms of healthy fats. Fats make up sixty percent of the brain and the nerves that run every system in your body. So, the healthier the fats in your diet, the healthier your brain. Omega-3 fatty acids, specifically the DHA component, are the top fat for brain development and function, immune response, heart health, and joint health, just to name a few. Omega-3s are essential fatty acids that affect every cell in your body, and the only way to get them is through food or supplements. Increased omega-3 intake has been linked to enhanced memory function and less oxidative stress, which will help keep your "mommy brain" clear.

If your baby is receiving breastmilk, then Baby will also benefit from the omega-3s in your diet (some pediatricians will even test your milk for omega-3 levels). Brain growth occurs most rapidly during the first year of life—an infant's brain triples in size by their first birthday. Fifty percent of the calories in mother's milk are from fat, so it's important that this fat is healthy.

Aim for 1000 milligrams of DHA in your daily diet. Here are some foods that can help boost your intake:

- Omega-3 enriched eggs
- Rainbow trout
- Albacore (or white) canned tuna
- Wild Alaskan salmon
- Flaxseeds
- Chia seeds
- Walnuts
- Soybeans
- High-quality omega-3 supplement

Lemon-Turmeric-Honey Salmon

2 (6-ounce) fresh or defrosted fillets
   of wild Alaskan salmon
1 teaspoon dried thyme
½ teaspoon turmeric
   Pinch of sea salt
   Pinch of crushed red pepper (optional)
1 tablespoon honey
2 slices lemon
1 tablespoon olive oil
   Pinch of black pepper

Preheat the oven to 375°F.

Place the salmon fillets in a glass baking dish.

In a small bowl, combine salt, olive oil, thyme, honey, turmeric, black pepper, and crushed red pepper (if using) and pour over the salmon. Place one lemon slice on each fillet.

Bake the fillets for 10–15 minutes. Be careful not to overcook.

Note: Always season to taste. If you like spicy food, and it doesn't bother your baby, use the red pepper.

Also, instead of baking the salmon, you can sauté it: cook the salmon in the oil and seasoning mixture in a skillet over medium heat for four minutes. Turn the fillets, top each fillet with one lemon slice and cook for four more minutes.

Serves 2

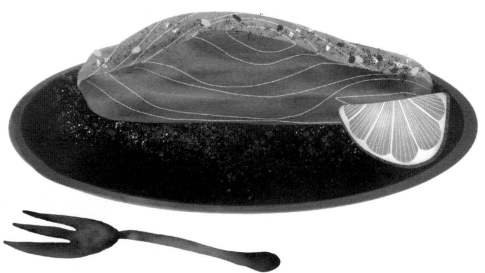

HOUSEHOLD BALANCE

"A mother's work is never done." This common saying reflects the experience of moms everywhere. While it carries truth, it also has the potential to overwhelm and rob you of joy and greatly hinder your mothering experience. Some moms find it very difficult to enjoy quality time with their babies or to take time for self-care when there are chores left undone. Finding household balance will likely be an ongoing journey. It's helpful to remember to prioritize the important—and not always the urgent. You may need to practice giving yourself permission to leave a sink full of dirty dishes or laundry unfolded in order to catch a much-needed cat nap or to sit and eat a proper meal. Remember, this is only a season; there will come a day when other household responsibilities can have a more primary role.

What do you and your family want to remember most from this season? When you look back at pictures, will you notice the clutter or the smiles? Remember that *your* mental, emotional, and physical well-being matters more than that of your household.

I have fifteen minutes of "hands-free" time; what do I do?

_____

_____

_____

How do I feel about how my household is currently being
run? What, if anything, is out of balance?

_____

_____

_____

How do I feel about the division of labor? How can I communicate
with my partner about this to avoid resentment?

_____

_____

What can I delegate or let go of so that I can focus on my priorities?

_____

_____

_____

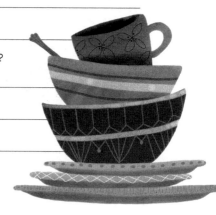

Are household finances a source of tension? How am I managing that?

_____

_____

In what ways do I keep from getting overwhelmed by my household responsibilities?

_____

_____

This is what I want my family to remember most about our family's home life:

_____

_____

TO PONDER

How are aspects of my childhood showing up in how I run my household?
How do my partner's attitude and energy affect
my ability to find household balance?

A MOMENT FOR ME
Finding Balance

As a job, being a mom is full of physical, mental, emotional, and financial demands, and it can easily lead to stress. This is where balance comes in. Here are ideas for balancing work, household responsibilities, and some mama time.

Do a childcare swap with a friend. Take turns watching each other's baby while the other mom has some free time. Use that hour or two to do whatever gives you the most peace. The kiddos like the play time with each other also!

Join a gym that has reputable childcare.

Find a moms group that offers childcare support (MOPS offers free childcare during the meeting).

Find a carrier that Baby likes and explore different ways of wearing Baby. When they are big enough to look out over the top, many babies love the backpack style. This is a fantastic way to have two hands free for household duties.

Don't be afraid to let your partner, friends, and family help. Find an activity that your partner can commit to doing with Baby once a week, like story time at the local library or a trip to the park. Having activities like this built into your household rhythm is the perfect step toward balance.

BACK TO WORK

Going back to work after Baby comes can be a huge challenge for new moms to navigate. Some moms may be eager to get back to their day jobs, while others can't imagine having the capacity to reengage with their careers—and many moms feel a bit of both. While work situations and demands vastly vary, most come with an array of complex emotions. There can be a sense of relief from allowing another to take over the care of your baby for a chunk of time. Yet with that relief may come some "mom guilt." Some moms report feeling panic and dread at the thought of leaving Baby even for a few hours. And some moms have the luxury of choosing whether or not to hold a day job while others do not—which brings its own set of complex feelings. Whether you're going back to work full time, part time, or are embracing your new job as a stay-at-home mom, the transition back to work should be met with incredible self-acceptance, tons of patience, and the knowledge that you are doing your best for your family.

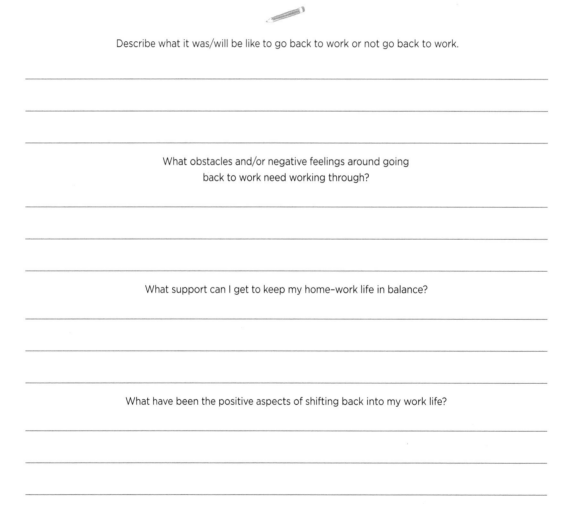

Describe what it was/will be like to go back to work or not go back to work.

_____

_____

_____

What obstacles and/or negative feelings around going
back to work need working through?

_____

_____

What support can I get to keep my home–work life in balance?

_____

_____

What have been the positive aspects of shifting back into my work life?

_____

_____

_____

In what ways do I anticipate having to shift my work arrangements
to fit the needs of my new family situation?

_____

_____

_____

_____

_____

How will my mothering experience enrich my work life, and vice versa?

_____

_____

_____

_____

TO PONDER

Is there something about my work situation that is causing
resentment? What is in my control to change?
Do I see my baby as a disruption of my work life, or my
work life as a disruption of my family life?

A MOMENT FOR ME
Affirmation for Returning to Work

If others can do it, so can I. I will treasure the precious time I have at home with my baby. I am becoming stronger because of this challenge. I am setting an example of a loving and hard-working mother. I am showing my little one that working hard for one's passions and goals is admirable. I surround my heart with compassion as I make tough decisions, while I simply do my best one day at a time.

Final Reflections

Cleaning your house while your kids are still growing is
like shoveling the walk before it stops snowing.

ERMA BOMBECK

How does the reality of this quote make me feel as I
envision the future of my new family life?

_____

_____

_____

_____

What did becoming a mother teach me or show me about myself
recently? How can I carry this lesson throughout my life?

_____

_____

_____

_____

What have I read, watched, or listened to recently that I want to remember?

_____

_____

_____

What worries or fears about motherhood have I been able to work through?

_____

_____

_____

_____

What thoughts can I be mindful of that decrease my joy and peace, and
how can I best work through them and, if needed, get support?

_____

_____

_____

_____

How have I surprised myself or made myself proud as a mother?

_____

_____

_____

What do I want to let go of that is not serving me well?

_____

_____

_____

What would my future self want to say to me right now?

_____

_____

_____

A commitment, declaration, intention, or promise to myself moving forward
that helps me hold tight to what I have learned in this chapter:

_____

_____

_____

_____

A Love Note to Myself

Take some time to truly appreciate all that you are and all that you do for yourself, your baby, and those around you. Celebrate YOU in writing and memorialize the parts of yourself that deserve love and acknowledgment. Return to your words from time to time when you need a reminder.

Dear Me,

_____

_____

_____

_____

_____

_____

_____

_____

_____

_____

_____

_____

_____

_____

Draw, doodle, or attach pictures that describe
the essence of you becoming a mother.

9

FAMILY BONDING

A rich family life depends on creating and sustaining emotional bonds through shared family connections, traditions, and celebrations. Sharing values and a sense of identity, along with establishing clear and healthy boundaries, is an invaluable aspect of being a family unit. But a clear sense of values, identity, and boundaries doesn't happen automatically or overnight. It is a journey, and the process unfolds over time. You are just starting to build the framework that will support your family. There will be setbacks, restarts, and recalibrations. Right now, you get to dream and envision what you want for your family.

When you take time to establish family bonds, it gives your family an opportunity to see your heart, the true essence of who you are, and not just your busy, half-distracted way of operating. It sends the clear message that you are thinking about and acting on what is truly important. When a family is bonded, the inevitable stressors and frustrations of this world are easier to take in stride. These meaningful bonds provide stability and a sense of well-being that will sustain you and replenish you.

Fancy vacations, lavish birthday parties, and keeping up with the latest tech trends might add excitement and adventure, but often it is the simplest moments, however small, that build strong family bonds, which no amount of money can provide. Our job, then, is to be present often enough to recognize and make the most of those golden moments. If you're like many women and are an avid multi-tasker who is used to being in at least two places at once, this may take some practice. But you will be pleasantly surprised at the joy and fulfillment that these magical moments bring.

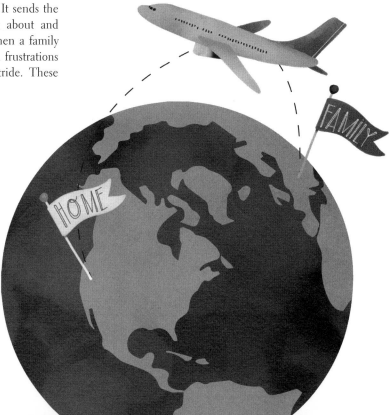

You don't choose your family. They are
God's gift to you as you are to them.

DESMOND TUTU

In what ways do I see myself as a divine gift to my family?

_____

_____

_____

_____

_____

_____

_____

_____

_____

_____

_____

_____

_____

_____

_____

FOSTERING CONNECTION

Connectedness is the mutual emotional bond between people that lasts over time and fosters an ongoing sense of belonging and security. Feeling connected is thought to be the most important factor in a family's ultimate success and happiness. For mothers whose relationship with their own parents was not a close one, connecting with their baby can be a source of emotional healing and provide a new trajectory for their own family. While for some this connection may happen naturally and spontaneously, most moms find that they must be intentional about it amidst all that is vying for their attention. By nurturing your relationships with your partner and children, you are creating the most important bonds of your life. And you are teaching your children, no matter how young they are, how to relate to the world around them—all while making memories that will last a lifetime.

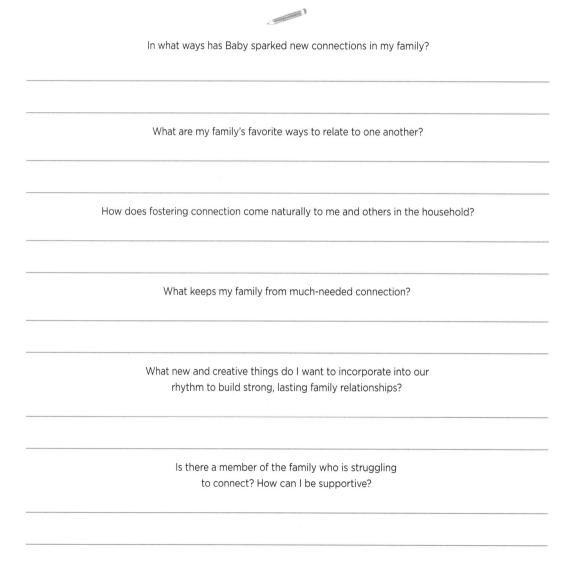

In what ways has Baby sparked new connections in my family?

_____

_____

What are my family's favorite ways to relate to one another?

_____

_____

How does fostering connection come naturally to me and others in the household?

_____

_____

What keeps my family from much-needed connection?

_____

_____

What new and creative things do I want to incorporate into our
rhythm to build strong, lasting family relationships?

_____

_____

Is there a member of the family who is struggling
to connect? How can I be supportive?

_____

_____

How has being a mother been a source of healing for
me? How about for others in my household?

TO PONDER

In what ways has becoming a mother allowed me
to connect to myself in a deeper way?
Do I feel capable of fostering the connection I desire in my
family, or do I need to get some guidance and support?

A MOMENT FOR ME
Staying Connected and Charged

"You can't pour from an empty cup." This old saying is simple yet apt when it comes to connection and being present for your family. Staying in tune with yourself is essential. Many moms also find it comforting, and even necessary, to connect to a source bigger than or outside of themselves.

Here are some tips for recharging your spiritual batteries:

UPON AWAKENING What is the first thought in your head? Set a simple intention or say a quote or prayer. For example: "God, I put my day in your hands." If the association with God doesn't resonate with you, then simply replace that name with someone or something that does.

CONNECT THROUGH RELATIONSHIPS Have you ever heard the expression "Be God with skin on"? It describes how we might show grace to others through our actions and connect with those who

send that grace and love back to us. Most of us have a number of human encounters each day, some of which are uplifting and some deflating. Connecting through relationships can be as simple as reaching out to a friend who may be struggling, or going on a walk with someone who makes you smile. Keeping our spiritual battery at a healthy level allows a softer, more tolerant mindset to guide our more challenging encounters.

MINDFUL BREATHING Set a timer for five minutes. Start in a quiet, comfortable place and read a paragraph or two from an inspirational book. This helps focus the mind. Close your eyes and tune in to how you're feeling. Acknowledge your thoughts and feelings without judgment, and then visualize them leaving your mental and physical space. Breathing slow and steady through your nose, inhale for four counts, hold for two counts, exhale for four counts, and hold for two counts. Repeat. Imagine a soft, calm energy on the inhale and a deep sense of connection on the exhale.

FAMILY TRADITIONS AND CELEBRATIONS

Family traditions and celebrations are among the best ways to nurture family connection. Traditions can be stories, rituals, beliefs, and customs that your family maintains and passes on from generation to generation. They give family members a sense of unity and infuse the world with meaning. Traditions and celebrations help keep us grounded and focused on family heritage and important family beliefs. Whether we're celebrating holidays, birthdays, milestones, or accomplishments, traditions give us the opportunity to live together in the moment and enjoy something that we have created as a family. They also give us a chance to slow down, appreciate, and express gratitude for our family's culture and history. Simply the anticipation of these special moments can bring a childlike joy to the household that your children will notice and embrace. If traditions and celebrations were not a part of your childhood, this is the perfect time for your family to start creating their own.

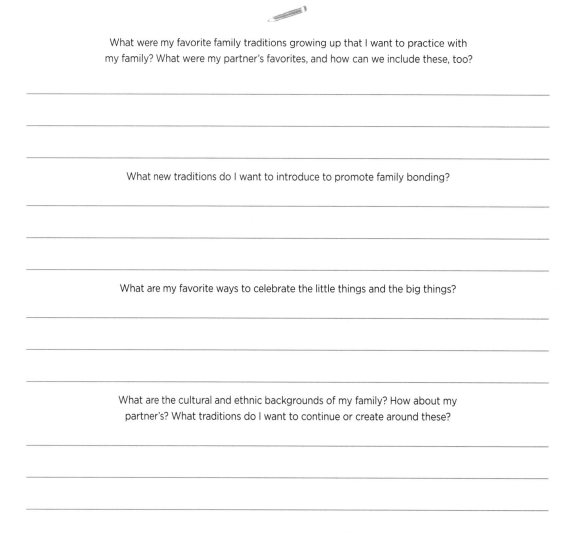

What were my favorite family traditions growing up that I want to practice with my family? What were my partner's favorites, and how can we include these, too?

_____

_____

_____

What new traditions do I want to introduce to promote family bonding?

_____

_____

_____

What are my favorite ways to celebrate the little things and the big things?

_____

_____

_____

What are the cultural and ethnic backgrounds of my family? How about my partner's? What traditions do I want to continue or create around these?

_____

_____

_____

Are there any painful memories associated with holidays or traditions from your childhood that need to be worked through? How about your partner?

_____

_____

_____

Are there any traditions or celebrations around my religious beliefs or spiritual practices that are important to teach my child?

_____

_____

TO PONDER

Is there something that is keeping me from
leaning into intentional celebration?
Is there a holiday or tradition that I felt was not
complete without a child of my own?

A MOMENT FOR ME
Mom Squad Traditions

Perhaps you are more outgoing and festive than the rest of your family. Connecting with your closest friends, a.k.a. your mom squad, is another great way to honor the traditions that are important to you. Remember, your mom squad is a part of your tribe, so find ways to celebrate with them! Here are some ideas:

Take turns hosting holiday activities like a
    pumpkin patch or Christmas cookie decorating
Do an annual secret-sister gift exchange
Organize a book club that meets
    monthly or bimonthly
Commit to taking a moms' night
    out at least once a month
Do a simple craft project together

Write in some more options for your mom squad:

_____

_____

_____

_____

_____

Self-Care Check In

On a scale of 1 to 10, where 1 means "really struggling" and 10 means "no problem":

What is my current stress level?

1   2   3   4   5   6   7   8   9   10

What is my current level of joy?

1   2   3   4   5   6   7   8   9   10

How am I doing on my self-talk/thought life?

1   2   3   4   5   6   7   8   9   10

Am I making nutrition and hydration a priority?

1   2   3   4   5   6   7   8   9   10

Am I managing my mental health?

1   2   3   4   5   6   7   8   9   10

Am I getting enough sleep and rest?

1   2   3   4   5   6   7   8   9   10

How am I doing at staying present?

1   2   3   4   5   6   7   8   9   10

Am I being supported in my mothering?

1   2   3   4   5   6   7   8   9   10

Am I making enough space for myself and my needs?

1   2   3   4   5   6   7   8   9   10

NOURISHMENT TIP
Fruit

Fruit is an important source of many nutrients, including potassium, fiber, vitamin C, and folate. It is also a great way to satisfy your sweet tooth and get much-needed energy for mom life! It's recommended that we eat five servings per day. Use your fist as a guide: one fistful equals one serving. Over the course of a day, five servings might look like this:

- ½ cup of organic blueberries added to oatmeal

- 1 small banana and ½ cup of strawberries in a smoothie (counts for two servings)

- 1 medium apple, sliced, with nut butter

- Baked pear recipe (see right) for dessert, or Greek yogurt and fruit of choice

Baked Pear with Dried Cranberries and Greek Yogurt

1 Bosc pear, halved and cored
1 tablespoon organic virgin coconut oil, melted
   Cinnamon to taste
½ cup plain, unsweetened Greek yogurt
2 tablespoons unsweetened dried cranberries
2–4 tablespoons pistachios
   Raw honey (or coconut palm sugar)

Preheat the oven to 400°F.

Place the pear halves in a glass baking dish. Drizzle with the melted coconut oil and sprinkle with cinnamon.

Bake to the desired softness, 30–40 minutes. Top with the yogurt and pistachios and lightly drizzle with honey.

Serves 2

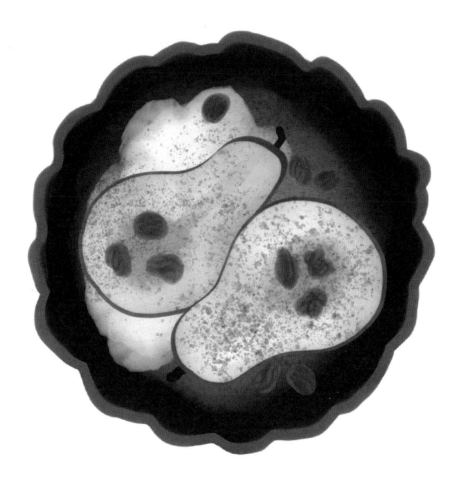

BOUNDARIES

Establishing clear, healthy boundaries helps family dynamics stay in balance. Personal boundaries are the physical, emotional, and mental limits we establish to protect our hearts, our time, and our well-being. They enable us to separate who we are, and what we think and feel, from the thoughts and feelings of others. At the same time, they teach those around us what is okay and what is not okay. Holding boundaries is one way of communicating to others (and ourselves) that we have value and self-respect. With only so much of ourselves to go around, we must know when to say no in order to say yes to what is important. If you too often find yourself drained or resentful, this is a clue that you may not be upholding clear boundaries. The good news is that your new role as Mom gives you a perfect opportunity to establish or reevaluate your boundaries, making sure they align with what you want for yourself and your family.

Below is a list of the most common areas around which a mom must establish clear boundaries. Take some time to assess where you're at with each one and how you can bring healthier balance, if needed.

Social media: _____

_____

_____

Screen time: _____

_____

Work/career: _____

_____

Finances: _____

_____

Food, beverages, and nutrition: _____

_____

Friendships: _____

_____

Extended family: _____

_____

Partner: _____

_____

Baby: _____

_____

Other: _____

_____

TO PONDER

Does setting and holding boundaries come naturally
to me, or does it take effort and intention?
How would it feel to live and structure my life around healthy
boundaries? How might doing this make me feel more free?

A MOMENT FOR ME
Nighttime Restoration

Whew! You made it through another day. Congratulations! Maybe boundaries were a challenge, or maybe the little one had a particularly needy day and all you want to do is clock out. We see you. While there is definitely a time and place for shutting your brain off with Netflix, here are some more restorative practices to consider as you unwind.

Take an Epsom salts bath with
    peppermint essential oils
Crochet or enjoy an adult coloring book to
    give your hands a relaxing and creative
    outlet other than mindless snacking
Try some restorative yoga poses
Write a gratitude list
Enjoy a cup of tea and a great book
Record your thoughts in this journal!

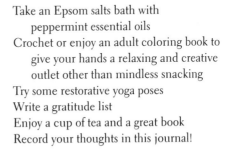

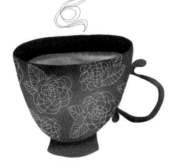

FAMILY MISSION STATEMENT

Creating a family mission statement is a great way to foster family bonding around specific, shared values. It can be hard to narrow down which values you most want your family to emulate (because we want everything for our children!). But it's important to clearly decide what you want your family to be known for over time. "We are a family that . . . (shows respect, is honest, is loyal, has faith, practices gratitude, is generous, travels together, plays sports, serves, invests in education, etc.)." This shared family identity—stated, reinforced, and celebrated—will help your child naturally take on the virtues that are most valuable to you. Some day, your child will embrace her own standards and identity apart from you. But while she's young, your child will begin to learn what she stands for through your words, actions, and emotional interactions. It may feel like a lot of pressure knowing you are shaping your child's purpose and values. Allow this reality to excite and empower you! Be confident that wherever your family is currently, each day brings a new opportunity for growth, positive change, and the ability to rewrite your family's trajectory in the direction of the purpose you want to pursue. Stay focused on a growth mindset, knowing that intentionally creating your family's identity and mission statement is an ongoing process.

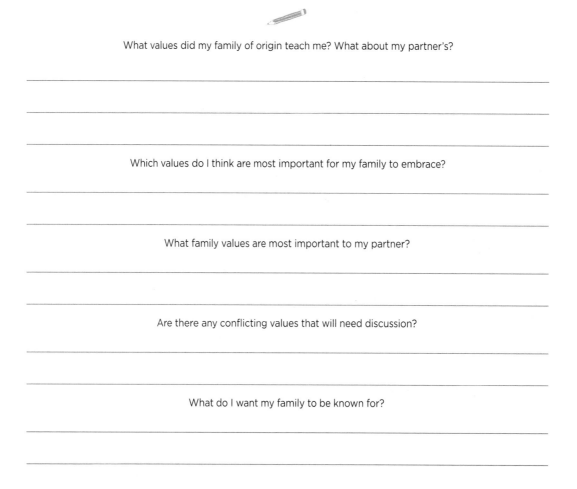

What values did my family of origin teach me? What about my partner's?

_____

_____

_____

Which values do I think are most important for my family to embrace?

_____

_____

What family values are most important to my partner?

_____

_____

Are there any conflicting values that will need discussion?

_____

_____

What do I want my family to be known for?

_____

_____

How am I currently teaching/fostering this legacy?

_____

_____

Do I have a strong sense of purpose? If so, what does that look
like, and how has it been shaped by becoming a mom?

_____

_____

My family mission statement: take a few minutes to put your thoughts together;
then, write a declarative statement of what you want for your family.

_____

_____

_____

_____

_____

_____

_____

_____

_____

_____

A MOMENT FOR ME
Mommy Mantra

I am called during this time to be a strong, compassionate woman and mama. I have everything inside of me to nurture myself and my family. I am focused on connecting within so I may be of maximum service to my family as we live out our mission statement. I dwell in a place of love, not fear. I will do my best, with the help of my partner and community, to embrace life and serve others as my energy allows. I wrap myself in compassion and grace as I navigate this wondrous new stage of life. I will laugh and love and live out my purpose. I am enough.

Final Reflections

*We will practice courage in our family by showing up, letting ourselves be
seen, and honoring vulnerability. We'll share our stories of struggle and
strength. There will always be room in our home for both. We will teach you
compassion by practicing compassion with ourselves first, then with each other.*

BRENÉ BROWN

What feelings came up when I wrote my family mission statement?
How does this make me think about my motherhood journey?

_____

_____

_____

_____

What did becoming a mother teach me or show me about myself
recently? How can I carry this lesson throughout my life?

_____

_____

_____

What have I read, watched, or listened to recently that I want to remember?

_____

_____

_____

What worries or fears about motherhood have I been able to work through?

_____

_____

_____

_____

What thoughts can I be mindful of that decrease my joy and peace, and
how can I best work through them and, if needed, get support?

_____

_____

_____

_____

How have I surprised myself or made myself proud as a mother?

_____

_____

_____

What do I want to let go of that is not serving me well?

_____

_____

_____

What would my future self want to say to me right now?

_____

_____

_____

A commitment, declaration, intention, or promise to myself moving forward
that helps me hold tight to what I have learned in this chapter:

_____

_____

_____

_____

A Love Note to Myself

Take some time to truly appreciate all that you are and all that you do for yourself, your baby, and those around you. Celebrate YOU in writing and memorialize the parts of yourself that deserve love and acknowledgment. Return to your words from time to time when you need a reminder.

Dear Me,

_____

_____

_____

_____

_____

_____

_____

_____

_____

_____

_____

_____

_____

_____

_____

Draw, doodle, or attach pictures that describe
the essence of you becoming a mother.

RECOMMENDED RESOURCES

Parenting

The Baby Book: Everything You Need to Know about Your Baby from Birth to Age Two by William Sears, MD, Martha Sears, RN, Robert Sears, MD, and James Sears, MD. Little, Brown, Revised Edition, 2013. America's bestselling "baby bible" and encyclopedic guide to the first two years of your baby's life.

The Attachment Parenting Book: A Commonsense Guide to Understanding and Nurturing Your Baby by William Sears, MD, and Martha Sears, RN. Little, Brown, 2011. America's foremost baby and childcare experts provide a practical and inspiring guide to connecting with your baby and the benefits of doing so early.

The Fussy Baby Book: Parenting Your High-Need Child from Birth to Age Five by William Sears, MD, and Martha Sears, RN. Little, Brown, 1996. Describes the characteristics of a "high-need" baby, suggests ways to soothe a fussy child, and discusses nutrition, discipline, and communication.

The Portable Pediatrician: Everything You Need to Know about Your Child's Health by William Sears, MD, Martha Sears, RN, Robert Sears, RN, James Sears, MD, and Peter Sears, MD. Little, Brown, 2011. Invaluable information on common childhood illnesses and emergencies, including when to call the doctor, reassuring signs that your child is okay, and how to treat your child at home—all in a convenient A-to-Z format.

The Baby Sleep Book: The Complete Guide to a Good Night's Rest for the Whole Family by William Sears, MD, Martha Sears, RN, Robert Sears, MD, and James Sears, MD. Little, Brown, 2005. A comprehensive, reassuring, solution-filled sleep resource that every family will want to own.

25 Things Every New Mom Should Know: Essential First Steps for Mothers by Martha Sears, RN, with William Sears, MD. Harvard Common Press, 2017. Some aspects of mothering come naturally; others do not. This book offers insightful tips and helps new moms gain perspective as they transition into their new roles.

25 Things Every New Dad Should Know: Essential First Steps for Fathers by Robert Sears, MD, and James Sears, MD. Harvard Common Press, 2017. This book shows new dads what to expect so they can support their families and get the most out of the amazing newborn journey.

Becoming a Father: How to Nurture & Enjoy Your Family (The Growing Family Series) by William Sears, MD. La Leche League International, 2003. A collection of Dr. Bill's tips on being the best dad you can be.

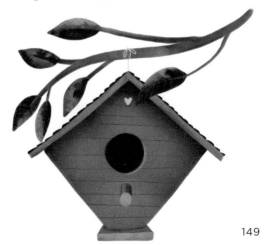

Attachment Parenting International (API), attachmentparenting.org.
This network of experienced parents offers essential tools, resources, and support groups for those interested in the attachment parenting philosophy.

"Postpartum Depression Facts," National Institute of Mental Health.
As a new parent, it may be difficult to know if what you're feeling is sleep deprivation, baby blues, or postpartum depression. Read more on postpartum depression and what to do if you think you have it at nimh.nih.gov/health/publications/postpartum-depressionfacts/index.shtml.

Babywearing International, babywearinginternational.org.
This nonprofit provides free, educational meetings to help you find the best carrier for your baby and lifestyle.

Arm's Reach Co-Sleeper, armsreach.com.
A bedside bassinet that enables baby and mother to safely sleep close to each other for easier nighttime comforting and feeding.

Breastfeeding

The Breastfeeding Book: Everything You Need to Know about Nursing Your Child from Birth Through Weaning by Martha Sears, RN, and William Sears, MD. Little, Brown, 2018.
Comprehensive, reassuring, authoritative information on many aspects of breastfeeding and weaning.

La Leche League International (LLLI), lalecheleague.org.
The most experienced and trusted resource and support group for breastfeeding mothers.

Nutrition

The Dr. Sears T5 Wellness Plan: Transform Your Mind and Body, Five Changes in Five Weeks by William Sears, MD, and Erin Sears Basile, MA. BenBella Books, Inc., 2017.
This five-step, five-week mind and body makeover—field-tested by the authors in their medical and health-coaching practices—changes your body's biochemistry to help you feel better, look better, and enjoy the new you.

The Family Nutrition Book: Everything You Need to Know About Feeding Your Children—From Birth Through Adolescence by William Sears, MD, and Martha Sears, RN. Little, Brown, 1999.
This book presents a comprehensive health plan called L.E.A.N., which stands for lifestyle, exercise, attitude, and nutrition, the four keys to optimal health.

Dr. Sears Wellness Institute, drsearswellnessinstitute.org.
Online interactive workshops that teach parents the best health and nutrition habits for their family's well-being.

ABOUT THE AUTHORS

Martha Sears

Martha is a registered nurse, former childbirth educator, La Leche League leader, lactation consultant, and most recently, coauthor of *The Healthy Pregnancy Journal*. With renowned pediatrician William Sears, MD, Martha is the coauthor of more than twenty-five parenting books drawing on her experience with their eight children (including Stephen, who has Down syndrome, and Lauren, their adopted daughter). She contributes to the content of askdrsears.com and is noted for her advice on how to handle the most common problems facing today's mothers with their changing lifestyles. Martha lives in Southern California and is blessed to spend tons of time with her grandchildren. She enjoys reading, gardening, sailing, and ballroom dancing with her husband.

Hayden Sears Darnell

Hayden, mother of three, is a certified health and nutrition coach who loves helping families and individuals on their journey toward better health. She is the coauthor of *The Healthy Pregnancy Journal* and contributing author to *The Healthy Brain Book*. The oldest daughter of Dr. William and Martha Sears, she has worked with the Sears Family Pediatrics medical practice for over fifteen years as Wellness Coordinator. She is a featured writer for askdrsears.com; has been a guest on TV shows and news stations sharing nutrition tips, healthy meal options, and the benefits of baby wearing; and co-hosted *The Dr. Sears Family Podcast*. Hayden owns a Juice Plus+ virtual franchise and travels all over the world speaking about how to keep ourselves and our families healthy. She received her MA from Azusa Pacific University and resides in Southern California. Having homeschooled for ten years, she now volunteers at her kids' schools and enjoys dancing, performing arts, and yoga.

Erin Sears Basile

Erin, first-time mom, is a certified health and wellness coach, yoga teacher, fitness instructor, and published author. Through her own health transformation, she quickly caught the health and fitness bug and is honored to help others find their passion for health. She is a featured writer for askdrsears.com and has been a guest on TV shows and podcasts including *Hallmark's Home and Family*, *The Dr. Nandi Show*, and *Just Jenny*. She holds an MA in music from Azusa Pacific University, a Master Health Coach certification from The Dr. Sears Wellness Institute, and multiple fitness certifications. In addition to her fitness work, she teaches voice and piano lessons, owns a Juice Plus+ virtual franchise and a health and wellness coaching business, and is coauthor of *The Dr. Sears T5 Wellness Plan*. She encourages and guides her students to live a joyful, connected life one day at a time.

ABOUT SOUNDS TRUE

Sounds True is a multimedia publisher whose mission is to inspire and support personal transformation and spiritual awakening. Founded in 1985 and located in Boulder, Colorado, we work with many of the leading spiritual teachers, thinkers, healers, and visionary artists of our time. We strive with every title to preserve the essential "living wisdom" of the author or artist. It is our goal to create products that not only provide information to a reader or listener but also embody the quality of a wisdom transmission.

For those seeking genuine transformation, Sounds True is your trusted partner. At SoundsTrue.com you will find a wealth of free resources to support your journey, including exclusive weekly audio interviews, free downloads, interactive learning tools, and other special savings on all our titles.

To learn more, please visit SoundsTrue.com/freegifts or call us toll-free at 800.333.9185.

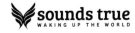